More Than a Health Cri

More Than a Health Crisis

Securitization and the US Response to the 2013–2016 Ebola Outbreak

Jessica Kirk

The MIT Press
Cambridge, Massachusetts
London, England

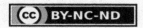
The MIT Press would like to thank the anonymous peer reviewers who provided comments on drafts of this book. The generous work of academic experts is essential for establishing the authority and quality of our publications. We acknowledge with gratitude the contributions of these otherwise uncredited readers.

This book was set in ITC Stone Serif Std and ITC Stone Sans Std by New Best-set Typesetters Ltd. Printed and bound in the United States of America.

Library of Congress Cataloging-in-Publication Data

Names: Kirk, Jessica, author.
Title: More than a health crisis : securitization and the US response to the
    2013–2016 Ebola outbreak / Jessica Kirk.
Other titles: Securitization and the US response to the 2013–2016 Ebola outbreak
Description: Cambridge, Massachusetts : The MIT Press, [2023] | Includes
    bibliographical references and index.
Identifiers: LCCN 2022052500 (print) | LCCN 2022052501 (ebook) |
    ISBN 9780262545693 (paperback) | ISBN 9780262374866 (epub) |
    ISBN 9780262374859 (pdf)
Subjects: MESH: Hemorrhagic Fever, Ebola | Security Measures | Disease Outbreaks |
    Global Health | United States
Classification: LCC RC140.5 (print) | LCC RC140.5 (ebook) | NLM WC 534 |
    DDC 616.9/18—dc23/eng/20230505
LC record available at https://lccn.loc.gov/2022052500
LC ebook record available at https://lccn.loc.gov/2022052501

10 9 8 7 6 5 4 3 2 1

To Mickael

Contents

Acknowledgments   ix
List of Abbreviations   xiii

1 Introduction   1
2 Setting Up Securitization   31
3 The Basic Securitizing Discourses   61
4 Securitizing Ebola   99
5 Securitizing beyond Ebola   135
6 Conclusion: Global Health beyond Ebola   163

Notes   179
References   181
Index   219

Acknowledgments

This book is based on my PhD dissertation, which in turn was based on a project completed during my master's degree. At each step of this journey, I have been immensely fortunate to have guidance and support from my stellar supervisors and mentors, my colleagues and friends, and my family.

The research for this book was mostly conducted during my PhD at the University of Queensland, where I was lucky to be under the supervision of Matt McDonald. I would not be here without Matt's guidance. This is more literal than one might think: he was the one who suggested I think about doing a PhD. Matt's support and help over the years of my program, continuing to this day, have been crucial, both in terms of his intellectual guidance (particularly in securitization theory and critical security studies but also in the more general areas of academic writing and research) and in the simple fact that I always knew Matt had my back. I owe him a debt I possibly can never repay. I also want to thank Shahar Hameiri for his associate supervision during this time. Shahar always gave me something to think about and question, and I am grateful for both that and his help in honing my final thesis.

Beyond my supervisory team, the School of Political Science and International Studies has provided an unparalleled supportive and enriching environment. Every person in this department is an inspiration; they are not only extraordinary scholars and staff but remarkable people, and the kindness they have shown me will remain with me always. Specifically, I want to note the generosity of Roland Bleiker. I asked Roland many years ago for some advice on research, and he has continued to this day to watch over my project and offer nuggets of wisdom. Equally crucial a part of this department were my fellow PhDs, who have shared my journey and allowed me to share theirs: Molly Murphy, Andrew Dougall, Josie Hornung,

Shannon Zimmerman, Larissa Hansford, Jan Phillip Mairhöfer, Cormac Opdebeeck Wilson, Paul Crawford, Jamal Nabulsi, Jack Shield, Megan Price, Federica Caso, Minh Vu, and many others. Each of these people has, at least at one point, had to put up with my need to blab incessantly about Ebola or securitization theory, my moments of crippling self-doubt, or my excessively loud "good mornings." Each aided in expanding my arguments, challenging them, and improving them. Each of them kept me sane, made me laugh, and made me feel a little less alone in this process. I consider you all an extended family.

I have been extremely fortunate to be able to conduct the work of translating my thesis into this book while holding a postdoctoral position in the Centre for Governance and Public Policy at Griffith University. In addition to the simple—but invaluable—support of a regular income, an office, and library access, Griffith has connected me to an amazing body of researchers in the School of Government and International Relations. In particular, I must single out Sara Davies for her amazing support. Sara is a fount of knowledge in more ways than one, and she is immensely generous with her time and insight. I have learned an enormous amount from working with her and I hope to continue to do so in the years to come. I also want to thank Cosmo Howard, Kai He, Diego Leiva, Lee Morgenbesser, Outi Donovan, Juliet Pietsch, Ferran Martinez i Coma, Xu Yi-chong, Louise O'Neil, and Angela MacDonald for their support and kindness during this period. Starting in a new department and revising a book during a pandemic is hard, but it has been made easier by said department being so supportive.

Beyond the institutions I've been a part of during this time, I am also appreciative of all the opportunities I have had to present my work, hear from key thinkers in my field, and discuss with brilliant minds. Arguments within this book have been presented to the International Political Studies Association World Congress, European International Studies Association Pan-European Conference, and Oceanic Conference on International Studies, where audiences have helped challenge and expand my arguments. I am also particularly thankful to some senior academics who have taken the time to discuss my work with me. Andrew Neal, Jeremy Youde, and Sophie Harman all gave me fantastic advice on conceptualizing security and global health security respectively, and the arguments in this book are stronger for it.

This book is very much a testament to the value of having strong relationships inside and outside academia. My "outside" friends, Irene Baker, Alex Carroll, Sammy Campbell, and Luke Osman, have helped me keep things in perspective and have been some of my greatest cheerleaders. Forgive me for disappearing so often into my work! My parents, Roly and Pam, perhaps never entirely understood why I "stayed at school" for so long, but their support has been unconditional and unwavering. I have been enormously lucky to always feel the warmth of their love and support, regardless of how far away I was and how often I failed to pick up the phone. I hope I make you both proud. Thank you also to my sister, Aimee, my nephew Malakai, and my nieces Siarra and Allaya, for always reminding me of what's important outside of my computer screen, books, and stacks of paper.

And the final, but most important, of my acknowledgments are to Mickael and Loki. Mickael, you are my best friend, my foundation, and the love of my life. This book would not have been possible without your love and support. And Loki, you are the goodest boy.

Jessica Kirk

April 2022

List of Abbreviations

AC360	*Anderson Cooper 360*
CDC	Centers for Disease Control and Prevention
CNN	Cable News Network
EB:O	*Erin Burnett: Outfront*
MSNBC	Microsoft National Broadcasting Company
NBC	National Broadcasting Company
NIH	National Institutes of Health
PN	Politics Nation
TOF	*The O'Reilly Factor*
UN	United Nations
USAID	United States Agency of International Development
WHO	World Health Organization

1 Introduction

In September 2014, as the outbreak of the Ebola Virus Disease (Ebola) in the West African states of Sierra Leone, Guinea, and Liberia approached sixty-five hundred cases, US President Barack Obama (2014d) declared that it was now "more than a health crisis", becoming a "threat to regional and global security." Citing the potential for "hundreds of thousands of people infected, with profound political and economic and security implications for all of us," Obama (2014b, 2014d) further designated the outbreak a "national security priority" for the US government and lobbied the UN and its member states to follow American leadership on the matter. In the wake of these proclamations, the US enacted a response that saw around three thousand Defense, USAID, and CDC workers sent to the affected states to join a civilian force of ten thousand people, while the US Congress eventually approved a $5.4 billion Ebola emergency fund, forming the largest American response to a global health emergency at that point in US history (until, of course, COVID-19) (White House 2015). This was despite the fact that, by September, the US homeland had experienced only the briefest of brushes with the outbreak in the isolated arrival and treatment of two health workers.

For many commentators, experts, and scholars observing these events this seemed a clear—and successful—instance of "securitization" (Burci 2014; Yanzhong 2014; McInnes 2016; Nunes 2016; Roemer-Mahler and Elbe 2016; Benton 2017; Honigsbaum 2017). Central to this idea is a rejection of "security" as objective and observable through mortality rates, scale of destruction, or any other indicator of "threat" (Wæver 1995; Buzan et al. 1998). This does not mean that these components are unimportant, but that they do not necessarily lead to an event being recognized as a security issue. "Security" is a label, constructed by political actors through discursively representing the issue as such. Applying this label to an issue is effectively to seek the dramatic elevation of its political significance, to ascribe to it particular meanings, and suggest particular, extraordinary responses over others. Success in this, however, is claimed to lie within its acceptance by a relevant audience, which permits "the breaking of rules" as a legitimate response. In other words, observers of the American response to Ebola have argued that Obama's labeling of Ebola as a security threat spoke not to an objective appreciation of danger but to a deeply political choice to enable an emergency response. For some, this was a welcome development; Ebola—in West Africa—*was* an emergency and demanded the kind of response that could only be justified with security (David L. Heymann, quoted in Horton 2017, 892). For others, however, this was worrying, potentially skewing the response away from the more mundane but vital public health measures needed (Burci 2014; Yanzhong 2014).

President Obama, of course, was not the only one "speaking security." American elites of various political persuasions, including both Republicans and Democrats, also labeled Ebola a threat and insisted an emergency response was required. Think tank experts, academics, and journalists fleshed out the details of both the outbreak and the disease itself, offering both reported facts and self-confessed conjecture. Twenty-four-hour news networks discussed new events in real time (and repeated frequently thereafter) both online and through television broadcasts. Indeed, from August 2014 to January 2015, the combination of these constant media reports, politicians' statements, and outside commentary led some to proclaim that the United States was suffering from an epidemic of "Fear-bola" (Petrow 2014; Robbins 2014). The securitization of Ebola was thus a public process, occurring at varying levels and involving a range of actors.

Yet this consensus over Ebola's "threatening" nature seemed to be the limit of agreement. Individual—but notable and vocal—politicians openly clashed across and within party lines over where the focus of the government should be, what response was most appropriate, and even what precisely the threat was. New Jersey Governor Chris Christie had a public war of words with both the White House and a nurse named Kaci Hickox over the appropriateness of quarantining health workers. While the president and various medical professionals urged calm (Obama 2014a; Dr. Thomas Frieden, in TSR 2014a), *Foreign Policy* magazine published an opinion piece from "global health expert" Laurie Garrett (2014b) proclaiming that

Americans were "not nearly scared enough about Ebola." And as CNN, ABC News, and other news outlets retraced the minute-by-minute movements of Craig Spencer, a doctor diagnosed as Ebola-positive in New York City (ABC News 2014; CBS News 2014; Newsroom 2014i), cable news pundits demanded the director of the CDC resign (Bill O'Reilly, in TOF 2014c) while opinion writers lamented the hysteria their colleagues were perpetuating (Blow 2014; Flanagin 2014b). Crucially, this rhetorical contestation had practical effect. State governors implemented quarantines despite the Obama administration and the CDC urging them not to. Businesses closed their doors, schools sent children and teachers home if they had traveled to (or had someone in their family travel to) anywhere in the continent of Africa, and flights were grounded, regardless of whether they directly linked to West Africa or not. Perhaps even more importantly, the positions of different actors also evolved. Obama (2014b, 2015), for instance, shifted from his initial September call to protect the "men and women and children [who] are just sitting, waiting to die, right now" to insisting, only six months later, that the US response was about "self-interest," "not charity." Practices also shifted: the government implemented enhanced airport screenings that a CDC review later suggested were merely to placate political opponents (Cohen et al. 2016, 58, 60). Ultimately, while Ebola did indeed seem to be securitized in the US, this was not a single, universally accepted utterance of security but a deeply debated clash of multiple, evolving claims to security.

This book asks two questions of this response. The first is why and how the Ebola outbreak in West Africa was securitized in the US. The outbreak did not objectively pose an existential threat to the US, so why was it represented as such and how was this successful? The second question delves deeper into this securitization, considering the contestation around it. How and why was the securitization of Ebola contested and what did this mean for the US response to the outbreak?

The foremost reason to ask these questions is simply that, so far, in-depth answers have been lacking. The existing global health security literature has certainly not ignored the Ebola outbreak, nor the role of securitization in the response. Indeed, analysis has aptly recognized the Ebola case as "an opportunity to consider anew the . . . relationship between health and security" (Enemark 2017a, 137). Contributions here have explored how the securitization of Ebola complicated efforts to allocate responsibility

(Wenham 2016), resulted in the absence of women and gender from discussions (Davies and Bennett 2016; Harman 2016), led to militarized responses with various benefits and problems (de Waal 2014; Kamradt-Scott et al. 2015; Benton 2017), prioritized short-term pharmaceutical solutions over longer-term health system building (Benton and Dionne 2015; Roemer-Mahler and Elbe 2016), revealed the flaws and priorities in global health governance (Fidler 2015; The Lancet 2015), and generally sparked a politics of fear (Nunes 2016). Some have also identified the existence of different understandings and approaches to security, considering how these were entwined with states' border control policies (Abeysinghe 2016), how domestic-level securitizations necessitated particular global responses (Enemark 2017a), and how the lack of engagement with a more humanitarian approach to health security complicated the response (Harman and Wenham 2018). Most of this analysis, however, has focused on the global response and/or specific components of the US response, such as quarantines (Hills 2016), media coverage (Seay and Dionne 2014; Russell 2016), and its tendency to treat West Africans as Others, or people who are inferior to 'us' (the Self) and thus less deserving of adequate treatment (Nunes 2016, 2017). There remains no detailed, in-depth, and careful examination of the US response to Ebola as a whole: how and why it was securitized, the contesting security narratives that existed within this securitization, and how this contestation affected the US response.

Yet the significance of this gap goes beyond its existence. Ultimately, this gap speaks to a wider one concerning American responses to global health emergencies. To understand this, we need only look to our most recent pandemic: COVID-19. Ebola and COVID-19 are undoubtedly distinct in key ways: unique epidemiological profiles (COVID-19 is a disease caused by SARS-CoV-2, a coronavirus, while Ebola is a hemorrhagic fever), vast differences in geographic spread (Ebola remained largely external to the US, while COVID-19 has caused a significant loss of American life), and significant variances in what was known and unknown about the disease at the time of its outbreak. Yet, despite these differences, there are also key similarities. The US response to COVID-19 involved experts and their expertise being dismissed and political authorities challenged. It led to enormous public debate over the appropriateness of particular measures, with these disputes grounded in claims of who is threatened (and who isn't), what exactly the threat is (and isn't), and what is known (and unknown) about the outbreak. It has also been thoroughly racialized, with the president of the United States insisting on referring to the virus by its country of origin and suggesting foreign Others were to blame for US travails. Much of the analysis of this has centered around the actions—and lack thereof—of this president and his fellow politicians (Altman 2020; Yong 2020), yet this cannot answer for why these disputes were even possible, much less successful, in undermining the response.

The Ebola case points to something deeper than the COVID-focused conclusions suggest, highlighting precedents and longer-running dynamics in the contemporary politics of health emergencies that are yet unanalyzed. If we are to truly understand how and why a powerful state actor like the US responds—and fails to respond—to a global health emergency like COVID-19, we need to delve deep into the politics of how disease outbreaks are understood by political elites and publics, how this intersects with wider political questions surrounding security and health (such as the role of experts in liberal democracies), what emergency actually looks like in practice, how each of these are contested, and how this contestation is dealt with (un)successfully. This book aims to provide such an in-depth examination, focusing on the Ebola response yet also offering a glimpse at the underlying politics of health security within the US.

In doing so, this book also contributes to our understanding of the wider securitization of disease and contemporary global health politics more generally. Specifically, this book focuses on domestic-level securitization: how a global health emergency is understood, debated, and responded to by and within a state. Although this has garnered some attention in journal articles, it has received less in-depth, book-length analysis, with global health security books tending to focus on the global. These books have provided considerable insight into global health governance (Harman 2012; Davies et al. 2015; Youde 2018a), international policy making (Hindmarch 2016), the rising prominence of surveillance and medical countermeasures (Fearnley 2008; Youde 2010; Elbe 2018), the shift toward preparedness (Lakoff 2017), or the general nexus between health and security (Davies 2010; Rushton 2019), but less on how and why crises are actually responded to by states in practice.[1] Why do powerful state responders like the US respond to distant health crises, and why do their responses take the forms that they do? Some claim that the label of "security" is necessary to garner their attention (and, more importantly, their resources), and enable particular practices (Elbe

2006; Youde 2018b). This book takes this idea and examines it in careful detail. How was the health-security nexus understood in a moment of crisis, the Ebola outbreak in 2014? What did this mean for practice?

This book is thus driven by the recognition that the US response to Ebola offers significant insight into the politics of global health emergencies. It engages these complex questions and provides detailed answers, thus offering a glimpse into what exactly happens when deadly microbes meet security. As a single case, it cannot, of course, generalize to provide a definitive statement on global health, Ebola, or COVID-19. Yet it can provide the kind of nuance, depth, and complexity that is currently missing from much of this analysis and seems to haunt our attempts to respond to new and more dangerous pathogens. It dives deep into the US response to Ebola, focusing specifically on the months between July 2014 and February 2015 and the public battle over how the outbreak was to be understood and responded to. It asks how exactly the outbreak of Ebola in West Africa was constructed as a security threat in the United States, moving away from the mere recognition that it was to consider the process by which this took place. It examines what underpinned this securitization: the values, concerns, knowledge, understandings of the world and the US's role within it, and security itself. It seeks, in other words, not only to describe how the Ebola outbreak in West Africa was securitized, but why and how this was possible.

The US Response to Ebola: An Overview

As mentioned, this book focuses on the US response to Ebola as it occurred during the months between July 2014 and February 2015. The outbreak, of course, extended beyond this period, as did efforts by the CDC, USAID, and the Department of Defense. Yet the bulk of the US response—and public debate—occurred during these months (see Figure 1.1). Moreover, as this book will demonstrate, this was the period in which the response was securitized. To provide some context for this analysis of securitization, however, let us first outline what exactly the outbreak and response consisted of.

Today it is widely believed that the outbreak in West Africa started in December 2013 with eighteen-month-old Emile Ouamouno in Guinea. From Emile, it spread to his mother, sister, grandmother, health care workers, attendees of the grandmother's funeral, and likely across the nearby borders into Sierra Leone and Liberia (Baize et al. 2014, 1422). On March

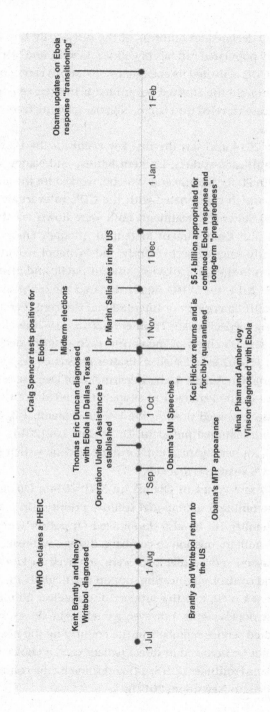

Figure 1.1

A timeline of key events in the US response.

23, 2014, the WHO declared an outbreak of the disease. By July 2014, all three of the densely populated capitals of Guinea, Liberia, and Sierra Leone had cases. The US CDC activated its emergency operations center on July 9, sending more staff to aid the affected governments in their responses. On July 20, a positive case traveled into Lagos, Nigeria, sparking fears of spread from the travel hub.

The end of July 2014 also saw the first key event for the US response. Two American health care workers, Dr. Kent Brantly and Nancy Writebol, were diagnosed with Ebola. Brantly and Writebol worked for the aid charity Samaritan's Purse, which coordinated with the CDC to evacuate the two back to the United States for treatment. Both were flown via the CDC's Aeromedical Biological Containment System to Atlanta's Emory University Hospital in early August. Both Brantly and Writebol would survive, but their evacuation to the US sparked significant public and media attention. On August 8, 2014, the WHO finally declared the outbreak in West Africa a Public Health Emergency of International Concern. For a number of critics—including Médecins Sans Frontières (2015, 11)—this timing was not coincidental. The US chiefs of mission in each country declared foreign disasters and USAID established a disaster assistance response team in Monrovia, Liberia. On August 5, the Department of Defense established an Ebola task force in the Pentagon to support this mission (JCOA 2016, 5). Yet the response remained slow. At the UN on September 2, Médecins Sans Frontières's international president, Dr. Joanne Liu (2014), made an unprecedented call for her organization: for states to deploy their militaries in assistance. The US answered that call.

September 2014 saw President Obama (in MTP 2014b; Obama 2014b; 2014d) declare the outbreak a "national security priority." In a speech to the CDC on September 16, he also announced Operation United Assistance, the first US military mission to combat a disease outbreak. Approximately three thousand service members were deployed to Liberia to aid with command and control, engineering support (particularly in constructing Ebola Treatment Units), logistics support, and medical training (JCOA 2016, 8–11). These deployments, however, would occur slowly, with only around four hundred service members in the country by the next month. They would also not be involved in direct patient care, a choice that frustrated Médecins Sans Frontières (2015, 14) and some media commentators (see Elizabeth Cohen, in Newsroom 2014f).

On the last day of September, a Liberian national named Thomas Eric Duncan was diagnosed with Ebola in Dallas, Texas. Duncan had begun experiencing symptoms on September 24 and went to Texas Health Presbyterian Hospital on September 25. They reportedly did not take his travel history, and sent him home with only a prescription for antibiotics. His condition worsened and Duncan returned to the same hospital on September 28 via ambulance, where his travel history was noted, an Ebola test taken, and the CDC notified. Duncan died on October 8, 2014. Two days later, one of the nurses who attended him—Nina Pham—reported a fever and went into isolation, testing positive on October 11. Another nurse, Amber Joy Vinson, tested positive on October 15, after having spent the weekend in Ohio.

Following this succession of events, calls were made by several media and political figures—notably Republicans such as Sen. Ted Cruz (2014a, 2014b)—for a ban on travel from West Africa. Obama (2014h) responded that such actions were unnecessary and even detrimental to the response. Instead, the CDC and Department of Homeland Security implemented "enhanced" airport screenings on October 8, a measure recognized by the CDC itself as politically motivated (Cohen et al. 2016, 58, 60). Calls were also made to fire CDC Director Frieden (Bill O'Reilly, in TOF 2014c), while Obama's seriousness about the response was called into question (Cruz 2014b). While the White House dismissed such claims, October 17 saw Ron Klain designated as the Ebola Response Coordinator or, as he was immediately known: the Ebola Czar.

By the end of October and early November, the debate on Ebola reached a fever pitch. Two events furthered this. One was the diagnosis on October 23 of Dr. Craig Spencer, a health worker returning from a deployment with Médecins Sans Frontières. Spencer had regularly checked for symptoms since returning and, while not displaying any, had traveled around New York visiting friends. Spencer was thus quickly framed by the media as a potential super-spreader (ABC News 2014; CBS News 2014; EB:O 2014f). In response to this apparent threat from returning health workers, the governors of New York (Andrew Cuomo) and New Jersey (Chris Christie) implemented mandatory twenty-one-day quarantines. The first day of these measures caught Kaci Hickox, a nurse returning from West Africa. Hickox did not take this quietly and mounted a media campaign and legal challenge against the quarantine. She was eventually allowed to return home.

The second key event which contributed to this heightened debate was the midterm elections, which occurred on November 4. While Ebola had been subject to partisan politics prior to these elections, the midterms saw Ebola this partisanship become explicit. Democrats and Republicans took positions on the Ebola response, namely the questions of quarantines and travel bans. In addition, Ebola was woven into a narrative of government incompetence, depicted as one of the four horsemen Obama was not protecting the American people from (Parker 2014). Republicans gained their largest majority in the Senate and the House of Representatives in decades. Following the midterm elections, Obama (2014k) requested an additional $6.18 billion in "emergency appropriations" for Ebola, framed in terms of his "foremost priority . . . to protect the health and safety of Americans" and "prevent additional cases at home." Notably, this included the creation of domestic Ebola treatment centers. This request was largely ($5.4 billion) approved in December.

After this point, however, attention to Ebola dropped. In fact, it dropped so dramatically that some feared the response would follow (Ban 2014; Coons 2015). The outbreak had hit its peak and was now slowing but not yet under control. A series of logistical, organizational, and staffing delays meant that this was also the point at which US-built treatment units opened (JCOA 2016, 51). Efforts in West Africa continued with little public attention within the US, until February 11, 2015, when Obama (2015) announced a "transitioning" of the response, including the return of all but one hundred of the troops stationed in Liberia. While he stressed that "America's work is not done" and some—namely the CDC, USAID, and some members of the military—would remain in West Africa, this was now a "civilian response." This response would end only in 2016, when each of the three states was finally Ebola-free. Nearly three years after Emile Ouamouno died, the outbreak ended with more than 11,325 deaths.

This is a necessarily brief overview of the US response. It is also one that focuses almost exclusively on what happened, bypassing the questions of *how* and *why*. Such an overview aids us in understanding what the response looked like, but it cannot answer of the questions outlined in the opening of this book: Why was Ebola responded to as a security threat? How and why was this label contested and what did this mean for the response? One might notice from this overview little discussion of security. Yet ideas of security infused each of these moments, including the silence and closure at the end. As new events occurred, competing ideas of Ebola's danger gave them competing meanings, clashing on key questions of what the threat was and whom it threatened. The response shifted in accordance, prioritizing efforts to save West Africans at one point and seeking to track their infected bodies as potential threats at the next. We must therefore add to our understanding of what happened an exploration of the how. In essence, this overview provides a scaffolding for the subsequent analysis: the key events that will be given substance through our analysis of securitization.

Global Health Security and the Securitization of Disease

Ebola, of course, was not securitized out of nowhere, nor without precedent. Indeed, for some, the securitization of Ebola was "déjà vu" (Roemer-Mahler and Elbe 2016, 489), with Ebola yet another disease outbreak—after HIV/ AIDS, SARS, H5N1, and H1N1—placed in the realm of security. Previous linkages between disease and security—embodied in the increasingly influential concept of *global health security*—created a context wherein Ebola's representation as a security threat was plausible and informed just how Ebola could be securitized.

Yet global health security and the health-security nexus more broadly remain debated. Multiple and competing understandings of health security exist, branching from differing depictions of diseases as threats to security and competing ideas of how best to respond. These meanings are not all equal. The academic literature around global health security contains many diverse and critical perspectives, but real-world practices often hew more closely to a particular approach, one that reflects the interests and fears of the most powerful actors in global health governance. And even within this approach, variations appear in just how it manifests in relation to particular crises, diseases, and responses. These varied meanings—and the differing levels of power and influence they hold—infused the US Ebola response, fueling the different claims to security.

We can consider two broad umbrella approaches to health security: *human security* and *national security*. Human security conceptualizes security from the perspective of the individual, with security being a quality that individuals have or lack. Disease fits within such an understanding as both a direct and indirect threat. The presence of disease, of course, directly threatens an individual's life and wellbeing, with outbreaks threatening human security on a mass scale (Berlinguer 2003, Owen 2004, 347). Yet it is also an indirect harm, disrupting the positive feedback loop between health and economic security (Chen and Narasimham 2003, 41; Ogata and Sen 2003, 96; McInnes and Lee 2012, 143; Caballero-Anthony and Amul 2014, 35) and risking progress made in women's education and economic empowerment (Johnson and Garcia-Moreno 2003, 190–192; O'Manique and MacLean 2010, 467–472). Human security approaches to health security thus emphasize the individual as the referent object, disease as a direct and indirect threat (thus also drawing attention to pervasive structural vulnerabilities), and the need for more equitable global governance structures, further development, and the embrace of health as a human right to properly obtain health security.

National security, meanwhile, focuses on the state as the referent object. The threat of disease, moreover, is not general (as a harm in of itself) but specific: diseases are only threatening when they threaten the functions, interests, or existence of the state. They can threaten a state's military capabilities (Dupont 2001; Elbe 2002; Singer 2002), population (Elbe 2005; Price-Smith 2009, 11–12), vital systems and structures (Lakoff 2008), or its very existence (Ostergard 2002; Petersen 2002, 68; Price-Smith 2009, 89–114). Diseases can also be made into biological weapons and potentially used by other states or non-state actors (Kelle 2007; Koblentz 2009; Enemark 2014b). Notably, national security perspectives tend to conceptualize disease as an external threat, with diseases endemic to a state pushed into the realm of public health (Labonte and Gagnon 2010, 4–5, 16; Davies 2010, 15, 155). As Sara E. Davies (2010, 18–19) laments, this renders disease "a foreign enemy to be vanquished or contained" rather than a collective challenge.

This, of course, is not inclusive of every possible conceptualization of health security. The global health security literature, for instance, has outlined competing approaches, including a feminist approach (Wenham 2021) and those that view health security as emancipation (Nunes 2014b). Despite this plurality, however, the two broad approaches outlined above tend to dominate global health security as it is governed, institutionalized, and practiced (see Davies 2010), including in cases like the 2013–2016 Ebola outbreak. Or, more accurately, *one* of these two tends to dominate global health security, while the other operates as the most prominent alternative and critique. As several scholars have argued, global health security is predominantly *national* security in practice (Rushton 2011; 2019; McInnes and Lee 2012). Some have traced how the very concept itself is the direct result of a concerted—and enormously successful—state push to entrench national security discourses in global health governance bodies (King 2002; Davies 2008; Weir 2014). Specifically, it is the success of Western states, who have focused attention on diseases and health events that primarily affect them (infectious diseases, HIV/AIDS, bioterrorism) and obscured those that affect others (Rushton 2011, 780; Youde 2016, 162). This is not to suggest that human security understandings are entirely absent from global health security. Human security remains an influential alternative, a normative yardstick to which other understandings of disease as a security issue are compared. This is readily apparent within the Ebola literature, where the global response to Ebola was deemed an "epic failure" of what global health security should be (Fidler 2015), prioritizing "collective vulnerability" over "individual human security" and failing to recognize the unique insecurities of West Africans (The Lancet 2015; Caremel et al. 2017).

To explain this, many scholars have turned to *securitization theory*. Securitization theory offers a useful critical lens as it moves beyond the assumption that global health security is based on an objective *security-ness* to disease. It does not dispute that diseases are threatening, but its emphasis on security as an intersubjective construction shifts the analytical focus to how and why particular diseases are considered threatening in particular ways. Scholars here have highlighted that objective factors such as mortality and infection rates do not seem to correlate with securitization. Christian Enemark (2007, 1), for instance, argues that "the best candidates for securitization are those infectious disease threats that inspire particular human dread, and which therefore generate a level of societal disruption disproportionate to the mortality and morbidity they pose." Securitization also draws attention to the power politics at play, asking who is claiming (and heard to claim) security and where. Davies (2008) and Lorna Weir (2014), for instance, have pointed to the influence of Western (particularly American) infectious disease experts and state actors at the WHO during the creation of global health security. When the focus on the subjective nature of the securitization of disease is combined with the argument that these "threats" were constructed by Western states, the result is a more critical perspective on global health security, where it is indeed dominated by national security narratives, but not because these diseases are objectively threats to the state. Rather, this dominance is because this is how the security dimension of disease has been primarily constructed among powerful states, international organizations, and even select nongovernmental organizations. This explains why alternative conceptualizations of health security (such as human security) persist yet still lack significance.

In addition to providing this critical understanding of global health security as a whole, securitization theory enables a detailed examination of how real-world cases of the health-security nexus manifest. While national security perspectives may dominate at the macro level of global health security, they might not manifest in the same precise form in each case. Securitization theory's analytical emphasis on observing how threats are discursively constructed asks global health security scholars to trace just how a disease is securitized, by whom, to which audience, and to what effects. As Clare Wenham (2019, 1095) has noted, such a focus has revealed that "the meanings of both 'health' and 'security' . . . have varied depending on the immediate pathogen posing a threat." Securitization occurs differently depending on context, threat, actors, audience, and so on. The theory also encourages scholars to "inquir[e] into the political consequences of attaching health to a security signifier," focusing analyst attention on the "emergency measures"—new practices, the breaking of rules and norms, the expansion of state power—that result (Nunes 2014c, 64). Again, these manifest in different forms, such as military operations (Watterson and Kamradt-Scott 2016; Benton 2017; Guevara 2022, 18–19), the expansion of WHO authority (Hanrieder and Kreuder-Sonnen 2014), the intervention and transformation of other states (Hameiri and Jones 2015), and the governing and disciplining of specific ("risky") bodies within states (Elbe 2005, 407; Nunes 2014c, 64–66). The value of securitization, in other words, lies in its capacity to delve into the *political construction* of disease as a security threat and its consequences.

In essence, by considering the US response to Ebola as a case of securitization, we can critically engage the health-security nexus, including the major understandings of health security outlined above but, crucially, how they manifest (and change) in practice. The Ebola response was indeed entwined with global health security—the competing claims to security drew on those common to human security and national security, with the latter especially prominent—but this did not *determine* how the response played out. We must look to how precisely Ebola was represented as threatening, to whom, in what ways, to what effects, how this draws on established ideas of global health security, and how it transforms this concept further.

The US Securitization of Ebola

Ultimately, while Ebola was indeed securitized, this occurred not in a singular act, but through multiple and competing discourses. Discourses are "specific ensemble[s] of ideas, concepts, and categorizations that are produced, reproduced and transformed in a particular set of practices and through which meaning is given to physical and social realities" (Hajer 1995, 44). More than a single act, they are intersubjective systems of representation, spoken by multiple actors in multiple acts, through which the "truth" of an issue like Ebola is generated (and thus can be acted on). To speak of multiple and competing discourses, therefore, is to recognize that what the Ebola outbreak *was* and *meant* was never universally or objectively defined. Indeed, while each articulation adhered to the general representation of Ebola as a threat, the crucial details of this broad securitization differed dramatically. The threat itself was constructed in differing forms. Ebola was simultaneously a potential global pandemic with the possibility of mutation, an immediate existential threat to the people and states of West Africa, and a possible threat to the American people. Correspondingly, who or what was at risk varied: West African individuals competed for attention with the stability of their state, the American population, the global economy, and the very idea of *feeling secure*. Compounding these differences were similar divergences in who could be considered an authoritative actor, what and whose knowledge was valid, and what constituted an appropriate response. And the audiences of these securitizing moves changed, with some proclaiming themselves to be speaking on behalf of an understandably terrified public and others insisting that the American people were more rational and selfless than this suggested. These differing representations linked together to form broader ensembles that gave meaning to the outbreak and the US response. They were, essentially, *securitizing discourses*.

This book describes the US securitization of Ebola as a process of contestation between three securitizing discourses and one *counterdiscourse*, a term I use to describe a discourse that is not explicitly securitizing (nor desecuritizing) but serves to challenge the other discourses. The first, the Helpless

West Africa (HWA) discourse, invoked a human security-type understanding of the outbreak, representing the "helpless" West African as the referent object, in need of salvation from the Indispensable Nation of the US. The second, offered primarily by the Obama administration, is the Potential Global Catastrophe (PGC) discourse, which focused on the potential threat of spread to the somewhat nebulous referent object of "global stability" and linked this to US national security. And the last, but ultimately most prominent, securitizing discourse is one I label the America Under Threat (AUT) discourse. Here, the referent object of the securitizing discourse was the American populace, with the threat being the possible (hypothetical) spread of Ebola to the US homeland. Finally, an opposing discourse formed: the Fearbola counterdiscourse, which particularly challenged the AUT discourse (though it occasionally contested the other securitizing discourses as well) as an irrational and politicized understanding of the outbreak, one deserving of mockery and criticism.

These discourses did not merely exist in parallel. There were not multiple securitizations operating alongside or around one another. Rather, these discourses competed to define the "real" threat of Ebola and decide what the US—the government, the health system, the military, the media, and the public—should do in response. They challenged and complemented one another's representations while responding to challenges and alignments others provided. They—and the debate between them—shifted as a result. Certain representations and practices became untenable while others became necessary. Part of this can be explained by the events that played out, but only a very limited part. Each event was interpreted through the three securitizing discourses and counterdiscourse, sparking a battle over the "truth": both of the event itself and the wider significance for the outbreak and response. The diagnosis of Thomas Eric Duncan, for instance, was both evidence for the threat that West African travelers supposedly posed to the US and a reminder of the actual danger faced by those in West Africa. In essence, we cannot speak of the American securitization of Ebola without speaking of this process of construction and competition. The interplay of these securitizing discourses *was* the process of securitization.

Particular discourses were dominant at particular times, with the AUT discourse especially central when it counted: from September through November. Yet while this was the case, it is the space *between* the discourses where the US response outlined previously was formed, debated, and shifted. The enhanced airport screenings were introduced to respond to fears that the border was open, but demands for travel bans were rejected. Experimental drugs were provided to West Africa following a media debate over the ethics of using them on infected Westerners and not West Africans (Erin Burnett, in EB:O 2014e; Dionne 2014). Quarantines on health workers were implemented, both formally in some states (such as New Jersey and New York) and informally in others, and then lifted as representations of health workers (as threats and as heroes) competed. An Ebola Czar was introduced right at the moment the key expert authorities—namely CDC director Dr. Thomas Frieden—were being portrayed as incompetent political pawns. None of these actions—or the myriad smaller actions and repercussions of the debate—can be understood without exploring how different representations of threat, referent object, audience, knowledge, authority, and security interacted, contested, and complemented one another. *All* of the discourses and the interaction between them were politically consequential. Moreover, the discourses themselves shifted through this process, as they were reiterated and revised in response to these challenges and in order to interpret new events.

Accordingly, when I argue that the AUT discourse was dominant in this process of securitization, I do not mean that it was the single defining discourse of the debate or that it uniformly drove the US government's response. Rather, it *guided* this process of securitization. It narrowed the conditions of possibility for the debate (and thus the response), still allowing room for opposing discourses but setting the terms of this contestation. It reiterated key contextual discourses of the *outbreak narrative* (Wald 2008), the national security approach to global health security, and Africa as the Dark Continent, representing the US as threatened by the "diseased" African Other. It produced an accepting audience for their claims, articulating the American public as understandably afraid of the risk they (possibly) faced and clamoring for their leaders to protect them. Those asserting this discourse often presented themselves as those leaders, representing their opponents (including Obama) as failing in "the government's job" to protect their constituents (Chris Christie, in FNS 2014c). Crucially, they also undermined expert authority, representing figures such as CDC Director Frieden and NIAID Director Fauci as political puppets (not neutral experts) and highlighting the (unlikely) possibilities against the probabilities these experts focused on. And these claims were grounded in a traditional meaning of security—national security, the protection of the Self from the Other—merged with a logic of risk. The PGC, HWA, and Fearbola discourses shifted to either accommodate or challenge these representations, with the ultimate indicator of this being Obama's (2015) February assertion of the response as being "not charity" but "self-interest." Yet these successes also left the discourse unstable, as it was reproduced by competing approaches as immoral, political, opportunistic, irrational, speculative, and excessive. Particularly in the later stages of the debate, it was destabilized entirely, and this opened up space for competing discourses to come to prominence, allowing a shift in the latter stages of the response back toward West Africa. Yet even here the approaches emphasized their alignment to the AUT discourse.

Ultimately, at the center of the US securitization of Ebola—the multiple discourses, contestation, interplay, and AUT dominance—were key representations concerning the audience, authority, knowledge, security, and the Self versus the Other. The forms of these representations that dominated—the fearful American audience facing risk from the diseased West African Other, the benevolent political opposition utilizing "common sense" against the "politicized" experts and a "politically correct" president thinking more about "them" than "us", the prioritization of speculation and imaginative scenarios over probabilistic knowledge, and the traditional national security approach merged with risk—were also grounded in history and context beyond this single outbreak. They entwined with long-running domestic debates around US identity, its role in the world, and the position of the military in the US's global outreach They drew on prominent public perceptions of Africa (and Africans) as "dirty and diseased" (Seay and Dionne 2014). They reiterated dominant global health security concerns with infectious diseases and the need to contain them. They spoke to the tensions between the ideals of democratic politics as equal and open to the layperson and the reliance on expertise and technocrats in crisis decision-making, as well as the challenges to established knowledge emblematic of "post-truth" politics. And they reiterated a definition of security that, despite attempts to alter it for more humanitarian purposes, remains bound to the defense of the state against external threats. Yet these representations were never inevitable. The debate around them and divergences in competing discourses speak to the potential for different approaches and responses, and the shifts in policy over time and between actors demonstrate the capacity for these to inform practice.

This case thus attests to how central context and history are in securitizing outbreaks and even securitizing in general. Yet it also reveals how precarious this is: claims to securitize Ebola in this way were debated, disputed, and dismissed by certain actors—including those with the institutional power to act otherwise—during the entire period, and even when the response was guided and bound by this approach, challenges and divergences still existed. In essence, the US securitization of Ebola points to how we must not assume securitization—either that of disease or of any issue labeled "security"—occurs in a particular, static form or cannot be challenged or shift over time. We must be open to multiplicity, contestation, and change, and the role of history, context, and power within this process. This requires a particular approach to securitization theory, one that diverges from the original framework as outlined by its founding theorists: Barry Buzan, Ole Waever, and Jaap de Wilde (or the Copenhagen School).

Securitization and the Construction of Security

Securitization theory, in essence, argues that issues such as disease outbreaks are not perceived as security threats due to any objective danger they may pose but because they are *represented* as a threat to a receptive audience, which enables emergency measures that would otherwise not be permissible.[2] In its original formulation, the Copenhagen School operationalized this basic idea into an analytical framework. The basic framework (outlined in more detail in the next chapter) identifies a *securitizing actor* (a political authority, typically the sovereign or a speaker for the sovereign) who utters a *securitizing speech act*, which portrays an issue as an *existential threat* to a valued *referent object*. The acceptance of the threat by a *relevant audience* endorses *emergency measures* "beyond the rules that would otherwise bind" (Buzan et al. 1998, 5).

While this is the basic, original framework of the Copenhagen School, it has been challenged, expanded, criticized, and reconceptualized by an enormous and diverse body of second-generation literature. Indeed, a more recent contribution to this work has argued that today, "there is no grand theory of securitization. Instead . . . there are various theories of securitization" (Balzacq et al. 2015, 517). These theories, despite their differences and debates, are bound together by "a common framework of thinking": the recognition that the successful claim to security transforms social reality, enabling those authorized to respond however they deem most appropriate (Balzacq et al. 2015, 518, 495). The core concepts—the securitizing actor, securitizing moves, referent object, audience, emergency measures—also remain, though the precise relationships between them (and weighting provided to each[3]) may differ depending on the approach. Some of these theories are often referred to as "schools"—such as the sociological school and the Paris School—while others are labeled according to their predominant ideological perspective (poststructuralist, neo-Marxist), yet even within these, significant variation occurs. Moreover, as Balzacq, Léonard, and Ruzicka (2015, 497) have aptly noted, there has been a notable amount of "cross-fertilization" between these schools and other approaches that risks being obscured should one adhere too strongly to labels.[4] The result is thus not multiple, completely distinct strands of securitization, but a broad "idea theory" of securitization that has inspired general approaches but still requires specific and more detailed "set up" for empirical analysis (Wæver 2011, 471).

This book therefore does not seek to offer yet another school or strand of securitization. Nor does it claim a significantly novel discovery about the theory, something that will shift the paradigm of securitization studies. Yet it also does not simply adopt one of the alternative frameworks of securitization, such as Balzacq's sociological model, and eschew all others. Rather, it considers just what securitization theory—both the general idea theory and the specific theoretical framework offered by the originating Copenhagen School—brings to the analysis of the US response to Ebola and, by extension, global health emergencies as a whole. It conducts a critical synthesis of the second-generation literature, exploring the critiques made, the alternative approaches offered, the limitations and benefits of each, and where these broad approaches clash and complement one another. Drawing from this work, it outlines a "set up" to analyze the contested, changing, and pluralized securitization of Ebola within the US, one that highlights context, the audience, multiple actors, knowledge, and the meanings and practices of security without rendering them static or singular. It is this empirical goal—rather than any a priori theoretical commitment to a particular model—that drives this book's examination of securitization theory.

Specifically, this book employs a conceptual framework that keeps the Copenhagen School's central focus on exceptionalism and security's meaning as sedimented but opens these concepts to (re)construction through discourse, including the possibility of multiple forms. The Copenhagen School, using Carl Schmitt's writings on *the exception*, considers security as exceptionalism: it places greater power in the hands of the sovereign, legitimates the breaking of rules and norms, produces "friends" and "enemies," and ruptures the normal political space. This is a valuable insight, highlighting the political effects of security, and it is well worth keeping. Yet, as Andrew W. Neal (2019) has aptly argued, this does not mean security is "anti-politics," particularly in its contemporary practice. Focusing on security as dichotomous to politics, as a complete break from the norm, denies an examination of how security is infused with normal politics, and how normal politics is infused with the politics of security in turn. This manifests in many of the issues highlighted by those typically categorized as part of the sociological school and the Paris School: the undertheorization of the audience and the lack of appreciation for context (Balzacq 2005; Stritzel 2007; Léonard and Kaunert 2010), the denial of multiple, professional, and non-elite actors (Bigo 2002; Doty 2007; Amoore and de Goede 2008), the refusal to consider different meanings or logics of security (Ciută 2009; McDonald 2012; Nunes 2014a, 2014b; Kirk 2020), and the overemphasis on extreme and illiberal emergency measures (Abrahamsen 2005; Aradau and van Munster 2008, 2011; Muller 2004; 2008). Efforts by these schools—as well as other approaches and the myriad ways they intersect—to rectify these gaps are thus efforts to repoliticize the security in securitization, to highlight its political *construction* in addition to its effects.

In line with this work, I move away from the single elite speech act to consider securitization as a process, one that considers how security is articulated over time, within contexts, between actors and audiences, and in what form. Yet, in order to analyze the US response to Ebola—with its multiple, competing, and changing claims to audience, authority, and context—it is important not to replace the static speech act explanation of securitization with an equally static explanation of securitization as determined by a purely objective enabling audience or context. Context, audience, authority, and power relations are crucial, but the US Ebola case problematizes the notion that they *decide* securitization success or failure.[5] Instead, there is a malleability or an *undecidability* to them; we should not consider them constructed entirely by securitizing claims, but they can receive new, competing, or shifting meanings. Within the US case, for instance, the representation of Africa as the Dark Continent took on multiple forms, used to justify both the claim that the US needed to intervene to save West Africans and the claim that *they* were the danger, their "backwardness" the source of the outbreak. Moreover, as Michael C. Williams (2010, 215) has aptly argued, such an approach also misses that the audience can be constructed through processes of securitization, as the claim to security and its practice can draw an awareness of the audience as an entity into existence. These disputes speak to some of the theoretical clashes within securitization studies, ultimately highlighting the need to consider which theoretical position works best in relation to our case.

I thus turn to a discursive approach to securitization. Specifically, I draw heavily from a discursive approach articulated by poststructuralist thinkers within securitization studies, as well as the supplements and challenges offered to this approach from neo-Marxist, Bourdieusian, and competing Foucauldian studies.[6] Rather than looking for a single elite speech act, this approach focuses on how security is intersubjectively constructed, examining articulations of security over time and across actors as securitizing discourse. It is, as David Campbell (1998, 5) describes it, an approach that "celebrates difference: the proliferation of perspectives, dimensions, and approaches to the very real dilemmas of global life." It focuses on how security is given meaning, whether in terms of threat, defense, protection, or wellbeing, and how security is practiced, including the extreme measures, the "little security nothings" (Huysmans 2011, 372), and the myriad practices in between that scholars of risk and the Paris School have identified as important (Bigo 2002; Amoore and de Goede 2005, 2008; de Goede and de Graaf 2013). It should be stressed that a discursive approach is not a linguistic approach to securitization, as is sometimes assumed. Discourses include practices. As Lene Hansen (2006, 19–20) argues, a discursive approach does not prioritize ideas above materiality. Rather, it examines the intersection of the two. Indeed, "neither ideas nor materiality have a meaningful presence separate from each other." An emphasis on discourse thus allows an exploration of context and the audience while not automatically ascribing to them a deterministic or causal role. It emphasizes practice and regimes of knowledge as vital parts of construction. And, importantly, it enables an analysis of change and contestation. Discourses are unstable, overlapping, and always in need of reiteration. This overlap and reiteration are where alteration, challenge, and dismissal—contestation, in other words—occur.

The contribution this book makes to the securitization literature is thus twofold. First, it furthers efforts to move beyond the original framework and its earlier alternatives to consider the ground between these starkly labeled strands of securitization. It is inspired by Balzacq, Léonard, and Ruzicka's (2015, 521) efforts to bridge approaches "that are often treated as key divides ("either/or") in the literature," with the fundamental aim being the empirical examination of the US response to Ebola. This book is thus in lively conversation with the second-generation literature rather than seeking to rewrite it, dismiss it, or compete with it. Second, it offers an in-depth analysis of contestation and multiplicity within securitization, particularly of how contesting discourses of security operate within a concrete case study. Again, the existence of contestation and multiplicity within securitization is not a novel insight, but this book offers a detailed examination of how such contestation and multiplicity manifest and operate in practice. These insights are grounded in this single case study, but they also speak to the wider dynamics of contestation and multiplicity within domestic-level securitization.

Studying the Securitization of Ebola

As the Copenhagen School itself has noted, analyzing securitization involves studying discourse (Buzan et al. 1998, 25). The conceptual framework outlined in this book sees securitization as a process in which securitizing discourses are articulated, rearticulated, enacted, and debated. Moreover, the foremost goal of this analysis is to capture the public debate about the outbreak and federal response and consider how it evolved through contestation over time. With all this in mind, the method of choice becomes clear: discourse analysis.

In general, discourse analysis involves observing the *systems of signification* that are discourses: their linkages of *signifiers* (or representations) and their differentiation against others to produce meaning around a central *dominant signifier*, the point where substitution cannot occur (Milliken 1999, 229; Doty 1996, 6–7). The basic task is therefore to identify these signifiers, or key representations, and analyze the relationships they have within this system. This involves identifying the dominant signifier, or the *nodal point* of the discourse, and the signifiers that are linked to it to provide meaning (Edkins 2002, 72). The original framework of securitization provides the basis for this: security is the dominant signifier, and the referent object, threat, security actor, audience, exception, and emergency measures are the linked signifiers that give this central signifier meaning. Drawing from work within more sociological variants of securitization, we also add constructions of contextual signifiers concerning history, identity, political systems and institutions, power relations, and so on. We then analyze the relationships between these signifiers. This involves examining the "positive process of linking" (for instance, emotional, motherly, reliant, and simple to give meaning to woman) and the "negative process of differentiation" (juxtaposition of these against those giving meaning to man) (Hansen 2006, 17). Importantly, as discourses are inherently unstable and always in need of maintenance, a crucial part of discourse analysis is examining the "play of practice," or how they are articulated and rearticulated, including how and where linkages and representations shift, change, and/ or disappear (Milliken 1999, 230).

Yet, as Lene Hansen (2006, 50–53) argues, applying this general method to foreign policy can take one of several approaches, focusing on different sets of actors, texts, and practices to grasp different aspects of meaning and practice making. I follow here her second foreign policy discourse model, the succinctly labeled "Model 2," which focuses on the "major actors and arenas" in foreign policy debates: the government, the opposition, and the news media (Hansen 2006, 54). Specifically, Model 2 involves analyzing the speeches, interviews, and statements of the government (here, the Obama Administration) and political opponents (Republicans and Democrats who disputed the party line), as well as congressional debates and the news reporting and commentary of these events (including the aforementioned speeches, interviews, and statements) within the media. It focuses on how official discourses are constructed, rearticulated, and/or challenged within these spaces and by these actors as well as which critical and/or opposing discourses are constructed, how prominent they become, and what role they play in the rearticulation of official discourses. The benefit of this approach is that it permits an exploration of government discourse and its power while not assuming it as hegemonic, and it focuses on public contestation and change with a particular emphasis on discourse (in)stability during ongoing crises. A potentially contentious decision here is not including social media as part of this exploration of public debate. Yet the significance of social media such as Twitter and Facebook is debatable; while it offers a way for "the audience" to engage more directly with politicians, experts, journalists, and one another, most of that engagement remains politically unremarkable and is even ignored by these actors. When it does become significant, through trending hashtags or viral posts for instance, it is often covered (and, crucially, [re]framed) by traditional media, who also increasingly use social media to canvas public opinion on "hot" issues such as Ebola. Accordingly, analyzing government, oppositional, and media texts captures the main arena for public debate surrounding the US response to Ebola while also touching on—and, one could argue, making politically relevant—wider public discourse.

Data gathering spanned across a number of sources. This included a variety of US government archives, news databases, and the websites of prominent political opponents (namely their press statements and archives of opinion pieces and blogs). The US government helpfully "freezes" the websites of its past administrations when a new one takes office, acting as an archive of all press materials, legislation, statements, fact sheets, and other content that these websites held. Specifically, I gathered transcripts of press conferences, addresses, speeches, statements, press releases, presidential proclamations, memoranda, and fact sheets from the archived Obama White House, State Department, Department of Defense, USAID, Department of Homeland Security, and CDC. I also consulted the Library of Congress and *Congressional Record* to gather transcripts of hearings, meetings, remarks, and introduced legislation. In addition, I gathered press conference transcripts for key events that were not captured by these sources. For instance, the announcement of Craig Spencer's diagnosis was made by the New York governor Andrew Cuomo and mayor Bill de Blasio. Prominent and relevant oppositional politicians were identified through congressional hearings, the *Congressional Record*, and media reporting, leading to a similar focus on their archived statements and media appearances. In order to be comprehensive, I gathered this data through exploring these online archives for the entire time period, selecting relevant materials through searching for the key term *Ebola* and relevant terms during specific events (the names of the infected, for instance). I cut this data down further through reading the remaining texts and selecting those that considered Ebola beyond a mere mention (listing it, for instance, as an issue among many).

The proliferation of media sources in the US context—and the shift away from common sources such as commercial television and newspapers

—means that analyzing media will be either inherently partial or far too expansive to be manageable. The goal in choosing media sources, accordingly, was to gauge different ideological and partisan perspectives and different formats of news coverage. Accordingly, I gathered reporting and commentary from the "Big Three" cable news channels (CNN, Fox News, and MSNBC, supplemented by NBC News) and three prominent nationwide newspapers (*USA Today, Washington Post*, and the *New York Times*) including their online articles. The TV channels were selected due to their national ratings (Fox News and CNN holding first and second place in cable news ratings), with the lower-rated MSNBC supplemented by its parent company NBC's news coverage to make up for this gap, and their capture of a useful spectrum of ideological and partisan positions. The newspapers were similarly chosen for their daily circulation, though the *Washington Post* was included for its extensive international reporting. I obtained media broadcast transcripts, online articles, and printed reports through the Factiva database. Again, I used the simple search term *Ebola* to find any and all mentions of the disease before selecting relevant articles and broadcast transcripts.

Analysis was conducted through a series of critical readings of these texts. In line with Hansen's Model 2, I focused first on the official discourse—the speeches, statements, interviews, and so on—of the Obama administration. I identified and listed the representations of Ebola and its threat that appeared: what the danger was represented as, who was represented as endangered, who the securitizing actors were (and why), who the audience was, and what the most appropriate response was. I highlighted those that were frequently rearticulated and I also noted the representations that linked to these securitizing representations: those of the US and its identity, those of West Africa and West Africans, those of other actors (public health experts, health workers, international organizations, opposing political figures), those of other issues deemed "security," security itself, and so on. As Hansen (2006, 37) aptly argues, it is not enough to simply identify the signs; we must analyze how they are linked, as it is here that meaning is produced and where meaning can be contested and undone. I used these as the basic "codes" in the program NVivo. Having outlined in broad strokes how the official discourse was constructed, I turned to the wider political sphere: oppositional politicians and the media. Within this first reading of these texts, I coded the transcripts through the codes identified previously, but also added to this list the common representations of Ebola, its threat, and the linked representations that appeared here. I also noted how the official discourse and its key representations were represented, rearticulated, challenged, and changed by these actors. From these readings, I also created a timeline of *key events*: "those situations where 'important facts' manifest themselves on the political and/or the media agenda and influence the official policy-identity constellation or force the official discourse to engage with political opposition and media criticism" (Hansen 2006, 28). This was compared to key moments of the US response as outlined by policy actors to observe where gaps and contradictions occurred. These first readings were thus to create a foundation: a general outline of the basic securitizing discourses and the initial contours of the public debate.

Subsequent readings expanded and deepened this initial reading, focusing specifically on the interplay between these discourses. Using the key events identified through the first reading and preliminary research on the US response, I traced how the government, opposition, and media represented Ebola, its threat, and the response around each event. What key representations were (re)articulated at each point (and by whom)? Which were challenged and diminished (and by whom)? How did the linkages and differentiations change, and how did this shift each securitizing discourse and, ultimately, the response itself? By reading through these texts myself, manually coding, and focusing on linkages and differentiations rather than relying simply on automated content analysis, I was able to identify nuances and contextual dependencies within the debate: where general terms like *security, risk, the American people*, and *Africa*, as well as specific figures (the president, experts such as CDC Director Frieden, notable Ebola sufferers such as Thomas Eric Duncan) were given slightly different meanings and where these meanings changed over time and between actors.

Book Outline

The first chapter of this book, titled "Setting Up Securitization," provides a comprehensive examination of its conceptual foundation: securitization theory. As outlined above, securitization is essential for analyzing the American response to Ebola, yet also requires some "set up" to do so adequately (Wæver 2011, 471). Securitization scholarship expands far beyond the founding Copenhagen School, with an enormous body of second-generation work expanding, critiquing, and reconceptualizing its theory and analytical framework. This chapter explores this work, focusing on what we should take from the Copenhagen School's approach and how the second-generation literature answers the limitations within it. In doing so, it ultimately sets up a discursive approach to securitization. This allows for multiple constructions of audience and the intersecting but not determinative role of context. It recognizes the structured power of actors but focuses on how they are authorized in processes of authorization. It acknowledges the "thickness" of the national security meaning of security, but also permits the possibility that it might be used in alternative ways. And it contains an expanded concept of exceptionalism, one that is not bound to the ideal of Carl Schmitt but considers variations of its key tenets, including those that might be labeled "risk." This, as I argue within this chapter, ultimately speaks to the continued validity of securitization theory but also hones it to better fulfill its core purpose: analyzing the politics of security.

The second and third chapters, "The Basic Securitizing Discourses" and "Securitizing Ebola," then apply this "set up" to the US response to the 2013–2016 Ebola outbreak in West Africa. "The Basic Securitizing Discourses" starts this analysis by considering how Ebola was variously securitized. It outlines the four basic discourses that were evident in the US process of securitization, with three securitizing discourses and one counterdiscourse. It maps these discourses, pointing to the key representations that constituted each claim to security: the threat Ebola proffered, the referent object in need of protection, the key securitizing actor that would do said protecting, what emergency measures were necessary to do this, who the audience was, and what "security" itself meant and did. It also highlights the contextual discourses that were entwined with each claim and shared between them. This focused analysis of the discourses, as I acknowledge, requires detaching each from the others, which risks diminishing the fact that each discourse was constructed, reiterated, and changed through its interactions with the other positions. Yet this allows a detailed examination of each discourse and, crucially, "identif[ies] the main convectors of discussion" between them (Hansen 2006, 84). As I argue in this chapter, this effectively produces an image of the debate's boundaries—the threats Ebola was claimed to make, the audiences spoken to, the authorities to be listened to, and the practices that were said to be required—and the conditions of possibility for the debate.

The subsequent chapter, "Securitizing Ebola," explores the space within these boundaries. Tracing their interaction through a chronological series of key events, this chapter provides a comprehensive overview of how the US securitization of Ebola played out. It focuses on the ways the basic securitizing discourses outlined in the preceding chapter clashed and shifted or reaffirmed themselves in this process. It thus allows an examination of the nuances, divergences, and evolution of each discourse as well as the key sites of contestation. Through this, I observe the rise of the AUT discourse, its impacts on the US response, the continued struggle of the PGC and HWA discourses against it, and the critical self-reflection through the Fearbola counterdiscourse that ultimately destabilized it. It is here, in other words, that the *process* of securitizing Ebola is illuminated and analyzed.

The fourth and final substantive chapter, "Securitizing beyond Ebola," draws this empirical analysis together. Here, I discuss the four key empirical findings about the US securitization of Ebola, moving beyond a discussion of how it was securitized to explore why this process took the form it did. In particular, this chapter highlights the entrenched discourses surrounding Africa as the Other, the contesting claims to authority and expertise (including the diminishment of medical expertise as authoritative), and the primacy of risk logics in defining the threat of Ebola. I also return to our consideration of the response as a whole, outlining how this contested process of securitization resulted in a response that was late, focused on containment, and in a form that neglected those who suffered the most. From this empirical basis, I then shift this discussion to focus on securitization itself. While the Ebola case cannot and should not be generalized to speak of securitization as a whole, it does provide new and interesting insights to our understanding of securitization as a contested process, namely in emphasizing the diversity (*and* sedimentation) of security's meaning and logic and the need for contextually grounded examinations.

The concluding chapter briefly revisits the main contentions of the book before moving the analysis up a level. Here, I focus on what this book provides to our understanding of global health security. I consider the insight it provides into the politics of expertise as they play out in global health emergencies, namely how expertise is ascribed and how it is contested. I affirm the value in analyzing health security as discourse, specifically its emphasis on the multiple and competing ways health security can be understood and practiced and the deeply domestic nature of health emergency response.

I also explore the securitization of disease as a whole, highlighting the central role of race, fear, and exceptionalism within this process. Finally, I bring these arguments to bear on the elephant in the room: COVID-19. As I outline here, the findings of this book cannot entirely answer for the COVID-19 response in the US. Differences between the outbreaks, the federal governments, and even public discourse mean easy equivalences cannot be drawn. Yet there are also a number of striking similarities between the two cases. Public health expertise has been debated, denied, and dismissed. Speculation has taken hold, with mainstream and social media (and some politicians) offering "knowledge" produced through "what ifs" and large-scale conspiracies. And debates persist over what security actually means and how disease outbreaks fit into these understandings. While this is firmly a book about Ebola, it still speaks to the wider politics of global health emergencies, particularly the messy role of context, the production of knowledge via speculation, and the politics of expertise. In fact, the main difference between COVID-19 and Ebola is that the latter speaks to a sadly more common tale: the suffering of distant Others turned into the fear of contagion for the self.

2 Setting Up Securitization

Introduction

As the book's introduction makes clear, the original Copenhagen School framework of securitization holds an almost contradictory position within this book. On the one hand, the theory of securitization is illuminative and valuable in analyzing both the politics of global health emergencies generally and the US response to Ebola specifically. Securitization theory's emphasis on security as intersubjectively constructed allows us to move away from questions of objective threat to consider how issues are linked to security and what the claim to security means for response. On the other hand, however, the original framework of securitization comes with a series of limitations that qualify this value and even potentially undermine analysis. This is not a novel insight. Indeed, there is a large body of second-generation securitization work that outlines the gaps within the original framework: the inability to capture alternative or evolving meanings of security, the undertheorization of context and the role of the audience, the lack of attention to securitizing actors beyond elites, and the absence of more bureaucratic, dispersed, and banal security practices. These limitations problematize efforts to properly identify and explain cases of securitization. They also—most importantly for our case—lead to an inability to capture multiplicity, contestation, and change in securitization processes , as each corresponds to a space where difference manifests.

Accordingly, we must turn to this wider, second-generation literature and its answers to these gaps for our analysis of Ebola. This does not call for the complete abandonment of the original Copenhagen School framework. Indeed, the framework remains insightful in key ways, namely in its base theory, its emphasis on security as constructed but also "thick" in meaning, and its understanding of security's logic as one of exceptionalism. Instead, we simply turn to those who have expanded, deepened, and supplemented this theory. A number of schools have formed around (or been retroactively connected to) the base theory—the sociological school being perhaps the most prominent, with the Paris School also notable—while alternatives based on theoretical commitments—such as poststructuralism, neo-Marxism, social constructivism, realism, and the work of Bourdieu and Goffman—have also flourished. For many contemporary scholars of securitization, these branches of securitization are now securitization itself, and employing the theory means committing to one of these distinct approaches. Yet, as Balzacq, Léonard, and Ruzicka (2015, 497) warn in their review of contemporary securitization studies, adhering rigidly to these categorizations may miss how these "strands" have "cross-fertilized over the years," particularly as they address similar problems and phenomena. Moreover, it obscures the variation within each broadly defined approach, as well as the diversity in scholars' positions. Some scholars bounce between schools or approaches. Some label themselves but are labeled by others differently. Describing the securitization literature in terms of rigid boundaries and uniformity within them is thus problematically partial. For analysis, adhering to a single approach at the outset is to limit one's work, which may be better served by arguments that derive from the spaces between these strands or from their overlap. It may even be disingenuous, as it will inevitably draw from other approaches without considering how these overlap and possibly clash.

This book is not driven by an a priori commitment to a particular approach to securitization. Rather, it is driven by a commitment to a particular puzzle within a particular case: understanding multiplicity, contestation, and change within the US response to Ebola. This chapter's role is to outline a conceptual framework that will facilitate this analysis. Rather than being structured by generalized theories of securitization, it focuses on the core components in need of consideration for this analysis: the audience, context, and securitizing actors and the meaning, logic, and practice of security itself. This allows an exploration of the various and competing ways these components of securitization have been conceptualized and analyzed as well as which approaches work best for this book's analysis of the Ebola response. In doing so, it follows Wæver's (2011, 471) advice to consider the basic theory of securitization as an "idea theory" and to "set up" a framework as one's empirical analysis demands.

The chapter thus commences with a basic outline of the original Copenhagen School framework of securitization and the key components to retain: its understanding of security as sedimented in meaning and exceptionalist in logic, its emphasis on intersubjective construction, and the basic concepts of securitizing actors, audiences, and emergency measures. I then turn to the second-generation securitization literature and its examination of the limitations outlined above: the undertheorization of the audience and context, the elite-centered speech act, and the static understanding of security's meaning and practice. I focus on each of these issues, drawing on the arguments made by the second-generation literature to outline how best to conceptualize the audience, context, actors, and the meaning and logic of security so as to enable my analysis of multiple and competing claims to security. As I argue here, this leads to an understanding of securitization as a process of discursive construction.

Indeed, this book ultimately takes a discursive approach to securitization. It is guided by the poststructuralist work within securitization studies, but also informed by its interactions with other critiques: the recognition of context and audience, bureaucratic fields, security's multiple meanings and the expansiveness of exceptionalism as a logic, and securitization as a process rather than a single speech act. It provides a critical synthesis of this work, one that is attuned to its limitations, blind spots, and metatheoretical commitments but also grounds and justifies them within the empirical case being examined. Moreover, this approach also recognizes the value of the original framework, namely its emphasis on exceptionalism and the relationship with normal politics. The final section of this chapter outlines this in detail, drawing the insights and critiques together to outline just how I employ securitization, from theory to practice.

Indeed, in a general sense, the underlying theme of the chapter is that the basic idea of securitization—security is constructed, accepted, and practiced on the basis of its discursive performance—is worth keeping. To a certain extent, this chapter serves as a defense of securitization theory, albeit one well acquainted with its flaws. More specifically, it accepts the criticism but, like the wider securitization literature, rejects that blanket dismissal is the only option. Instead, in line with this body of work, my goal here is to continue the discussion on how securitization theory can capture the diverse and contested politics of security, focusing specifically on the US response to Ebola.

Securitization, the Copenhagen Way

Securitization, as outlined by its founding Copenhagen School, refers broadly to a theory and an analytical framework. The theory is that which recognizes security "as a speech act" (Wæver 1995, 55), one which invokes a particular meaning and political logic. This means that "[b]y uttering 'security,' a state-representative moves a particular development into a specific area, and thereby claims a special right to use whatever means are necessary to block it" (Wæver 1995, 55). Threats are therefore not necessarily objectively threatening, but are constructed as such by the act of labeling it. This might suggest a relatively unlimited conception of security, but the Copenhagen School ascribes clear boundaries to this construction. More specifically, it observes security to have a *sedimented meaning* and a *logic of exceptionalism*.

In terms of the former, Wæver (1995, 47) outlines security's conceptual history, arguing that it reveals the concept to be bound to "a set of connotations that it cannot escape." Security's meaning within international relations has come to be, first and foremost, "about survival" (Buzan et al. 1998, 21). More specifically, it is oriented around *national* survival, the "survival of the unit as a basic political unit," and reproduces "the logic of war—of challenge-resistance (defense)-escalation-recognition/defeat" (Wæver 1995, 52–53). Despite how this sounds, the Copenhagen School does not objectivize security. On the contrary, it considers security as discursively constructed. The school simply claims that this construction has sedimented "as structure and become . . . so relatively stable that *one must do analysis on the basis that it continues*" (Buzan et al. 1998, 35, emphasis mine). Security may hold no objective meaning on its own, but a particular discourse—the realist tradition of national security—has sedimented over time and through repeated use to become our "reality" of the concept. In line with Felix Ciută (2009, 308), we can label this *the sedimentation argument*.

Meanwhile, as both Jef Huysmans (1998b) and Michael C. Williams (2003) have aptly highlighted, this sedimented meaning is paired with a logic of exceptionalism, one derived from the writings of Carl Schmitt

([1922] 2005, [1932] 2010). Schmitt observed genuine, authentic politics as those centered around the antagonistic relationship between "friend" and "enemy." This distinction unifies "the people" into a political collective (friend) under a representative sovereign, and gives this collective meaning (and the sovereign "authentic" purpose) through defining it against the enemy. This friend/enemy distinction reaches its most "political" when it has intensified to the point of the "real possibility" of mortal conflict and violent death (Huysmans 1998b, 580–581). The sovereign has sheer, absolute power, standing outside of a given legal or normative order and even able to suspend, dismiss, or replace it within this state of "exception" (Huysmans 1998b, 581–582). Schmitt's exceptionalism aligns almost exactly with securitization theory and its understanding of security. Security, for the Copenhagen School, is invoked through the identification of an existential threat (the threat of violent death) and relies on the creation of "mass identity" and "self-enforcing rivalries with other limited collectivities" (Buzan et al. 1998, 36–37; see also Wæver 1995, 64; Buzan and Wæver 2009, 256). Securitization theory also emphasizes the state of exception produced and legitimated by such claims, where the existential threat "lift[s an issue] above politics" so the sovereign can act without being bound by normal rules (Buzan et al. 1998, 26). The Copenhagen School, however, differs from Schmitt in one crucial sense: it considers this state of exception not "politics," but "security." Indeed, Wæver (2011, 478; 2015) has since acknowledged that securitization theory's understanding of security is Schmittian but insists that its conception of politics is instead Arendtian and must be *protected* from this encroachment of Schmittian exceptionalism. This is the core normative position of the theory (Wæver 1999, 334; Aradau 2004; Hansen 2012).

We can summarize the above as the theory of securitization: its conceptualization of security, its use, and its effects. From this foundation, the analytical framework of securitization—that which is employed by scholars to identify and analyze security—is built. This framework ultimately has three steps. First, an authoritative *securitizing actor* performs a *speech act*, portraying an issue as an existential threat to a *valued referent object* in what the Copenhagen School terms a *securitizing move*. The second step is *audience acceptance*: where "an audience" accepts that "something is an existential threat to a shared value" (Buzan et al. 1998, 31). The third, and final, step of securitization is the legitimization of *emergency measures*. Success is to be found within the ability of the actor to "break free of procedures or rules he or she would otherwise be bound by" (Buzan et al. 1998, 25).

Ultimately, using securitization theory, even if just through the basic framework, is to invoke a set of assumptions about security: its openness through the speech act, its historically bound meaning, and its exceptionalist underpinnings. The theory provides a series of important concepts: the securitizing actor, the audience, the valued referent object, and emergency measures. Together, these claims form what is widely recognized as a compelling and insightful perspective on security politics, highlighting its constructed nature, corrosive political effects, and the power both within and behind it. It is for these reasons that global health security scholars have used the theory so widely, including in analyzing the global Ebola response. And it is for these reasons that I consider the theory worth keeping.

Limitations and Gaps

Despite this value, however, this theory and framework also fail to account for the process through which Ebola was securitized in the US. To understand why and how, we must turn to the second generation of securitization scholarship, that which—like me—sees the theory as deeply insightful but also observe key limitations in its analytical promise.

First and foremost, the multiple claims to security evident within the US response are invisible within a framework that focuses exclusively on elite moments of speech and a rigidly narrow understanding of security. As outlined previously, the Copenhagen School conceptualizes security's meaning as sedimented and its logic as exceptionalism. With the former, security becomes limited to the national security approach, with speech acts identified not because they explicitly use the term *security* (which lacks precision, according to the Copenhagen School) but because they conform with the "grammar" of (national) security. As Ciută (2009, 310) has aptly argued, this effectively makes the securitization analyst the ultimate arbiter on whether a speech act is securitizing or not, overruling the securitizing actor's own intentions. It also means that claims to security that do not conform to this understanding (such as a claim to human security) are not observed as securitizing speech acts. However, as the wider securitization literature has demonstrated, these alternative claims are prevalent. Security's articulation can differ across geographic spaces and cultures (Bubandt

2005; Stritzel 2014), can change over time toward understandings more in line with risk (de Goede 2008; McInnes and Roemer-Mahler 2017), and will vary across sectors, such as environmental politics (Trombetta 2008) or scientific settings (Salter 2008b). Positive and progressive meanings of security can even exist and have a practical impact (Doty 1998; McDonald 2003). By conceptualizing security *solely* as being about survival and national security, the Copenhagen School misses this variation, including when it might appear alongside this traditional meaning, as within the US response to Ebola.

In addition, the Copenhagen School's use of Schmittian exceptionalism means an emphasis on the power of the sovereign to "decide" the exception and enact rule- and norm-breaking measures, resulting in an analytical focus on the speech of political elites. Yet, as a large number of second-generation scholars have demonstrated, political elites are not the only actors involved in securitization. Numerous scholars have pointed to the role of the media in securitizing, both that of news media in defining events as security concerns (O'Reilly 2008; Vultee 2010; Gray and Franck 2019) and popular media in crafting persuasive narratives of security (Weldes 1996; de Goede 2008; Muller 2008; Wald 2008). Scholars from the Paris School and risk studies have highlighted the role of "security professionals," including intelligence agencies, militaries, police, bureaucrats, surveillance providers, technical experts, and risk assessors, in deciding threats and measures, including through routine, everyday practices (Bigo 2002, 2014; Amoore and de Goede 2005, 2008). Even civilians have been shown to securitize, with Roxanne Lynn Doty (2007) and Mike Slaven (2021) both outlining how American citizens have been involved in securitizing immigration. By focusing exclusively on the political sovereign, these securitizing actors—and their claims to security—fall from analysis.

Emphasizing the Schmittian exception has impacts beyond elite-centrism. It also limits an analysis of how security is variously practiced and how this practice can be a site for contestation. For the Copenhagen School, emergency measures do not necessarily need to be implemented (recognizing this, perhaps, as too high a requirement), but there must be the capability to implement them. As Huysmans (1998b, 2011) and Williams (2003, 2011) have noted, this is essentially the idea that the invocation of security renders a "rupture" with normal (democratic) politics, centering power within the sovereign and permitting the breaking of legal, normative, and political restraints and even the creation of a new "norm." Yet, again, the second-generation literature reveals the flaws in this assumption. Security practice does not always occur in extreme, rule- or norm-breaking forms. The Paris School and work on risk have outlined how security operates not only through emergency measures but also within "the routines, the day-to-day practices, . . . the bureaucracies" (Bigo 2002, 73), such as border control (Neal 2009) and pandemic preparedness (Lakoff 2017; McInnes and Roemer-Mahler 2017; Kirk 2020). Notably, these insights have been applied to the (global) Ebola response, with Caremel et al. (2017, 80) arguing that the response demonstrated how "routines [are inseparable] from emergency response systems," forming a "government of exceptions" rather than a single, all-encompassing exception.

So far, these critiques have focused on the very existence of competing claims and practices of security. Yet even if we stretched the meaning and logic of security to include these variations, would securitization theory as outlined by the Copenhagen School be able to analyze contestation and change between them? Two more limitations of the original approach make such an analysis unlikely, even with an expanded concept of security. The first is the undertheorization of the sociological aspects of securitization, namely the audience and the role of context. The second (lurking beneath) is the analytical focus on the speech act rather than the process of securitization.

If we are to observe how multiple claims to security manifested, contested, and dominated/diminished, we need to be able to observe their wider social circumstances: how and why particular claims were constructed, were contested, were successful (or not), and/or changed. Yet the Copenhagen School offers little to analyze these social and contextual dynamics. The Copenhagen School approach—particularly as articulated within the 1998 book—emphasizes audience acceptance as indicative of success, which makes securitization intersubjective (Buzan et al. 1998, 31). Despite this apparent significance, however, who precisely the audience is, how and why it accepts particular securitizing moves, and how an analyst can identify it remain nebulous. No hints are offered by the Copenhagen School, leaving critics to argue that they view the audience as an "entity that simply accepts or rejects the interpretation of security put forward by the securitizing actor" or "agents without agency" (Côté 2016, 550; see also Balzacq 2010, 2; McDonald 2008, 572). A similar problem lies within the

Copenhagen School's understanding of context. The Copenhagen School mentions preexisting understandings of the threat and "facilitating conditions" for securitization (Buzan et al. 1998, 31–33), and their discussion of "sections," such as "military," "societal," and "environmental," recognizes that securitization differs across issue area (Buzan et al. 1998). Yet, as Matt McDonald (2008, 571–572) notes, these potential forms of engagement with context are given no analytical detail: the "facilitating conditions" are not actually part of the framework and the "sectors" do not seem to go further than simply recognizing difference across issue area.

For many critics within the second generation of securitization literature, this undertheorization of the audience and context is ultimately evidence of the larger problem: an overemphasis on the speech act over the process of securitization. Thierry Balzacq (2010, 1) argues that the Copenhagen School ultimately has a "linguistic" or "philosophical" reading of securitization, where "the conditions of possibility of threats are internal to the act of saying 'security.'" Holger Stritzel (2007, 377) similarly refers to the Copenhagen School's reading of securitization as an internalist one, which considers the speech act as "retroactively" constituting the social context. In other words, uttering "security" enacts security (and its context) in and of itself. Accordingly, the analytical focus lies on whether the speaker fulfilled the "felicity conditions" (or "conventional rules") of this speech act (threat, referent object, emergency measures), successfully constructing security. Meanwhile, the wider process of securitization—the construction of a threat that resonates with an audience, the power and authority of the speaker, audience acceptance, the enactment/acceptance of measures, and, of course, any possibility of contestation and change at any of these points—is lost.

For some, these issues are reasons to abandon securitization theory entirely and turn to other theoretical perspectives in our analysis (Jones 2011; Howell 2014). Yet securitization theory still provides significant insight. The basic idea of it—that security issues are constructed by securitizing actors, accepted by an audience, and enacted through emergency measures—remains the best way to understand the US response to Ebola, as evidenced by its continued usage (Burci 2014; Yanzhong 2014; McInnes 2016; Nunes 2016; Roemer-Mahler and Elbe 2016; Benton 2017; Honigsbaum 2017). The insights regarding the meaning of security as sedimented and the logic as one of exceptionalism are also valuable. We should recognize the historical sedimentation of the national security meaning, even as we deny that this petrified into an unassailable position as the *only* meaning. We must take the Copenhagen School's warnings regarding the power of security to disrupt normal democratic politics and enact exceptions, empowering political sovereigns and enabling the breaking of rules and norms. What we need is thus not to get rid of securitization, but to outline a "set up" that keeps these insights while answering for the limitations.

Revising Securitization

Fortunately, the second generation of securitization literature has already laid much of this path before us. In addition to highlighting these gaps and limitations, it has provided alternative models, entire schools of securitization, competing approaches to key concepts, and outside theories and concepts to supplement the gaps. Crucially, it has done so while also keeping what Wæver (2011, 470) has termed the *idea theory* of securitization: a "distinct concept at its centre" (securitization; security as constructed) and "key concepts [that] form a close integrated constellation" (securitizing actors, speech acts, audiences, emergency measures, etc). I thus draw heavily on this work, but I do so in a way that does not simply borrow one of the existing models. Nor do I pretend to offer a novel addition to this collection of approaches. Instead, I focus on the core problems that hinder my analysis of the US response to Ebola: the undertheorization of the audience, the lack of context, the elite-centrism, the narrow conceptualization of security's meaning and logic, and the need to consider securitization as a political process. Of course, all of these are ultimately intertwined, and I come into this theory-building with my own theoretical commitments. Yet I, like Balzacq, Léonard, and Ruzicka (2015, 497), see significant cross-fertilization between this second-generation work, and even as I do lean closer to one approach than others, this approach is supplemented by engagement with other perspectives. The goal here, in essence, is to take Wæver's (2011, 471) suggestion to "invest in theoretical work when doing empirical analysis" and construct a "set up"—"possibly with several theories and constructs for the occasion"—specifically to analyze the multiplicity, contestation, and change within the US Ebola response. I thus now outline the conceptual pieces that form this set up.

The Audience

In addressing the undertheorization of the audience, many second-generation securitization scholars turn to Balzacq (2005, 2010). For Balzacq (2010, 1–2), securitization must be understood as "a strategic (pragmatic) process that occurs within, and as a part of, a configuration of circumstances, including the context, the psycho-cultural disposition of the audience, and the power that both speaker and listener bring to the interaction." In essence, the audience must be *persuaded*; speech acts do not "do" anything in and of themselves but must resonate with the audience's "feelings, needs, and interests" (Balzacq 2010, 25–26). Even when the audience cannot immediately be seen, its "consequences are often visible" (Balzacq 2019, 336). In terms of analysis then, we must add to the basic framework of securitization an analysis of the audience's feelings, needs, and interests, their "psycho-cultural disposition," and the "degrees of continuity" between the audience and the speech act (Balzacq 2005, 174, 192; see also Stritzel 2014, 48). Stritzel (2007, 370) highlights the "positional power of actors," including the speaker-audience relationship. The key, in other words, is to outline the audience, its expectations, its position, and the securitizing move's *resonance* with them.

Such an approach is compelling. It brings the audience into analysis and focuses on just how they impact on securitization success. And from this foundation, securitization scholars have identified multiple and differing audiences. Mark Salter (2008b), adding Goffman's dramaturgical analysis, has outlined how various "settings" of securitizing moves exist, with distinct audiences (scientific, elite, technocratic, and popular, for instance). As he argues, "the audience is not always the public," and securitizing actors will tailor their speech in accordance with the setting in which they are speaking (Salter 2008b, 327–328). Paul Roe (2008) similarly points to how one audience (the general public) might reject a securitizing move while another, more structurally powerful one—the UK Parliament, for instance—will accept it, which enables emergency measures. Jocelyn Vaughn (2009) has also used this approach to demonstrate how securitizers can attempt to persuade multiple audiences with their claims, tailoring their articulations to appeal to each. As Juha A. Vuori (2008, 72) succinctly summarizes, the form of the security argument ultimately "depends on which audience it is directed at." Accordingly, analyzing securitizing moves should include a concurrent examination of who the move is aimed at, what kind of expectations they might have, what history and context they might draw on, and what symbols and emotional appeals would resonate with them.

Yet such work also has a worrying tendency to completely objectivize the audience. This is concerning for our case for two reasons. First, it runs the risk of "ontological gerrymandering," or the "manipulat[ion of] an analytic boundary to make certain phenomena problematic while leaving others unquestioned" (Miller and Holstein, quoted in Huysmans 1998b, 493–494). The meaning of threat may be constructed, but all else remains objective. This means that the analytical question of why securitization succeeds simply gets shifted to the "psycho-cultural disposition" or the "feelings, needs, and interests" of the audience (Balzacq 2005, 174, 192). Beyond potentially being ontologically contradictory, this approach cannot answer for how a single audience—such as "the American people" in the US Ebola response—can be understood in different ways, manifesting different securitizing claims and, crucially, change within these claims.

Secondly, and more importantly, this approach has the corrosive effect of diminishing the audience to a fixed variable rather than an interacting component within a social process. The possibility that the audience may interact in securitization in different ways—contesting claims, offering their own, suggesting change—is lost, as is the possibility that the audience's position in the process might change. Indeed, the audience itself may change: as Williams (2010, 215) points out, a securitizing move can create a receptive audience, not out of nothing but through "bringing it to consciousness of itself as a unified audience." Ultimately, the precise relationship between audiences, actors, and securitizing moves (and context, as will be discussed below) is simplified into a unidirectional one of cause and effect. Yet how can multiple, competing claims to security be possible if securitization is driven by the audience's static desires, interests, and needs? Multiple audiences may answer for this, but what if, as in the case of the US Ebola response, there are not clearly defined or separate audiences?

An alternative way of conceptualizing the audience in securitization may answer for this while also keeping the insights of this work: the existence of multiple audiences, the tailoring of speech acts to audiences, and the need to consider power dynamics and existing structures. This approach turns to the poststructuralist literature within the second generation of securitization scholarship. Specifically, Lene Hansen (2011) and Julie Wilhemsen (2017) have argued that the audience should be read through performativity. Performativity is normally acquainted with the work of Judith Butler (1990), who saw gender as performative in the sense that it is discursively constituted. It is through discourse that subject-positions are imposed on subjects (as gender norms are imposed on bodies), yet the subject also enacts, performs, and possibly internalizes this subjectivity (as people perform these gendered roles). Viewing the audience as performative is thus to see it as a subject-position, produced and performed within securitizing discourses "as a constituted subject whose 'opinion' might be detected through surveys, polls or elections," to which we can also add anecdotal claims, generalized descriptions, and any other form of representation that performs an identity and purpose (Hansen 2011, 360). This is not to claim that there are no individuals or groups listening or responding to securitizing claims, nor that responses (including overt claims to acceptance/rejection) are unimportant. Rather, it is to note that these individuals, groups, and responses become socially and politically important for securitization only when they "enter the discursive, political sphere" (Hansen 2011, 360–361). Plenty of (dis)agreement may occur among a populace, but relatively little of it enters the discursive sphere and the social reality it produces.

It may be illustrative to consider that all subjects are audiences in the basic sense that they listen to, respond to, and are affected by discourses, yet not all subjects are "the audience" of a securitizing move. It is the latter that is vital for securitization, both in terms of how it informs securitizing moves and how it corresponds to contestation. It allows us to focus critically on questions of who can speak and be known as "the audience" and who cannot and is silenced (see Hansen 2000). It directs us to consider the relationship between audiences and securitizing actors in more depth, as actors seek to produce "the audience" as their audience, the one they alone speak on behalf of. It also, crucially, permits audience agency, as individuals adopt the position of "audience member" and speak from it, including in letters to the editor, media vox pops, or in communication with their political representations. This moves away from the "speaker-audience" mode of communication to consider how "meaning and representation" are made "*between* a myriad of actors in society" (Wilhelmsen 2017, 166, emphasis mine).

This is a key site of contestation. There is never one single audience, but actors will suggest there is (and that they alone speak to/for it) in order to stabilize their own authority and undermine others. Indeed, actors may even be speaking to a specific audience (conservatives or Republican voters, for instance), but they will present this as *the* audience in order to close off or delegitimize others (and those who claim to speak for them). Of course, the inherent instability of discourse means that these constructions of the audience are always a site of contestation. In the US Ebola debate, for instance, Republicans frequently presented themselves as speaking for "the American people," who were frightened and demanding authoritative action, a demand that was being "ignored" by Obama. Obama, meanwhile, disputed this representation and suggested that Americans were instead rational, cosmopolitan in moral outlook, and sought to "fix problems" rather than running from them, a goal he shared and would achieve for them. These claims encompassed subject-positions of their opponents as speakers/security actors (Obama as eschewing his role as "voice of the people" and Republicans as fearmongering and counterproductive) but were ultimately centered on constructions of the audience.

Context

Context tends to be considered alongside audience by many second-generation scholars, both in their critiques and in their efforts to rectify this gap. Stritzel (2007, 367), for instance, considers the audience and context as part of an externalist reading of securitization to combat the Copenhagen School's internalist approach. This externalist reading views speech acts as "embedded" within a social context and examines securitizing moves in relation to actors' resources, power positions, and political struggles, the wider discursive background and history, and the processes of authorization in specific locations (Stritzel 2014, 44; see also McDonald 2008, 573). We must focus on the "sociolinguistic resources" used to "create resonance" (Stritzel 2014, 48), such as the "heuristic artefacts (metaphors, policy tools, image repertoires, analogies, stereotypes, emotions, etc.)" common to a context (Balzacq 2010, 3) or the bureaucratic "settings" actors and audiences see themselves within (Salter 2008b). We should also consider how securitizations are "translated" between contexts (Stritzel 2014), including the meaning of security itself (Bubandt 2005; Ciută 2009). In essence, we should indeed see securitizing moves as embedded within their social context and examine the alignment between the two. But how do we do this in a way that captures multiplicity, contestation, and change as needed to examine the US response to Ebola?

Again, we must be wary of ontological gerrymandering. Balzacq's suggestion to turn analytical focus to how security statements are "related to an external reality" (Balzacq 2010: 13), including the "brute threat" the issue might have (Balzacq 2005, 181), runs this risk. The reason ontological gerrymandering is so worrying here is that it tends to render context an immutable force with a deterministic role on securitization. Like objectivizing the audience, it renders context a single, static explanation for a security claim and its ostensible success. And again, the Ebola case shows the flaw in this assumption: the significance of context can differ and be a site of debate. Border security and immigration discourses (which claim that people were smuggling themselves into the US for better healthcare), for instance, were employed and had some level of success on some occasions, but they were also deeply controversial and *destabilized* security claims at other times. Similarly, Africa was represented as the Dark Continent, but this was presented in different ways: to justify helping the poor, passive West Africans, to keep the diseased peoples out and protect oneself, and to ensure that the rest of the world was not destabilized. Of course, this critique does not mean disputing the insights from this work entirely. Securitizing moves are not purely decided by an objective context, but actors work within it and must use the contextual resources at their disposal to craft their claims to security. Eric van Rythoven's (2021, 253) description of this process as "the field of claim-making" being shaped and constrained is an apt one and well worth adopting here.

To capture multiplicity while keeping the valuable emphasis on change and contestation, I further the emphasis on discourse apparent in such work. In fact, I expand this emphasis, moving away from approaches like critical discourse analysis, which sees discourse as "subordinate" to context (Stritzel 2014, 44), to one that considers context within discourse. Again, I turn to poststructuralist scholars. Despite some arguments to the contrary (Balzacq 2005, 180–181; Stritzel 2007, 360–362), poststructuralist discursive approaches do not diminish the role of context. As described by Doty (1996, 6), discourses are understood under poststructuralism to be unstable and to have "an overlapping quality," where their "exterior limits are constituted by other discourses that are themselves also open, inherently unstable, and always in the process of being articulated." This, as I will discuss, allows for multiple securitizing discourses and contestation between them. Importantly, it also allows for an examination of how context informs and is informed by contestation. The overlapping discourses include those that do not immediately pertain to the securitization of an issue but surround it, whether by being tangentially related to the issue (discourses of West Africa or Africans more generally) or connected to the practices involved (discourses surrounding the role of the US military). In other words, rather than a concrete, single "context," we consider the "relational site" of context (Campbell 1998, 221), or contextual discourses.

This does not return us to an internalist position, as some suggest. It considers securitizing claims as embedded in larger discourses that shape and constrain the "field of claim-making" (van Rythoven 2021, 253). Securitizing claims reiterate these discourses yet can also challenge and change them. As discourses are always unstable and in need of reiteration, context too shifts in its precise meaning and is reiterated in different ways. Thus general contextual discourses such as the Dark Continent or the Indispensable Nation took on varying forms, and others surrounding borders and immigration were disputed. Such an approach, in other words, allows us to explore the field of claim-making as a pluralized, contested arena.

Actors beyond Elites

As outlined in the discussion of the Copenhagen School's approach and its limitations, the elite-centrism of the Copenhagen School framework is largely due to its use of Schmittian exceptionalism and its emphasis on the political sovereign. Alterations to this approach to exceptionalism will be the focus of the next section, so let us focus for now on the more practical question of how to move beyond the securitizing elite to consider the wider array of possible securitizing actors. As Shahar Hameiri and Lee Jones (2015, 26) note, we should be careful not to replace the elite-centrism of the Copenhagen School with an equally restrictive focus solely on private actors, the media, or the "professionals of unease" outlined by the Paris School. Yet we also should not arbitrarily cut them from analysis or risk missing them as we focus on other actors.

Instead, we need to make self-reflexive decisions based on our empirical analysis. Where is securitization occurring? Which actors are visible (or potentially invisible) here and should be included? What is the interaction between these actors? These decisions will differ depending on one's case. Suzanne Hindmarch (2016), for instance, examines the securitization of HIV/AIDS as a policy process. In doing so, she maintains a focus on political elites at the first stage of "agenda setting" (which she connects to the Copenhagen School's speech act) and the second stage of the "framing contest" but expands to include bureaucratic actors in the third stage of this process ("policy implementation"). Such an approach works aptly for her case, where "abstract high-level policy directives" (the result of the first and second stages) move to "the bureaucratic processes required to implement these directives" (Hindmarch 2016, 27). Yet in the Ebola response, the rapid nature of the response meant that these steps were blended: responses were implemented as claims were made, and these were then contested and altered. Accordingly, the public "framing contests" that Hindmarch (2016, 26) observes in her second stage never ended. There is thus more analytical value for my case in considering how these responses and actors fed into such public contestation. This leads to a methodological choice, where I focus on those actors in the public discursive space: the media, political actors, experts, and policy practices as part of discourses. It also leads to a conceptual one, where I focus on how particular actors are authorized to securitize and practice security while others' authority is dismissed.

As Strizel (2014, 50–51) argues, securitization scholarship tends to assume the security actor's authority and assume it as stable. Such an assumption "should be replaced by the empirical study of processes of authorization." Some actors will hold positions of structural and institutional power. That may not necessarily translate into authority, however. We must therefore look to the discourse and the processes of authorization that occur within it. This includes questions of who is deemed worthy to speak, to be heard, and to be reiterated. Whose knowledge "counts" and why/why not? How is authority constructed and legitimated? What kinds of social capital are mobilized and in what ways? How is institutional power legitimized or delegitimized? With such a conceptual approach, we can observe both how elites are authorized (and their authority diminished) and how non-elites become security actors. Thus our analysis opens up to include experts or security professionals (as well as the media or politicians not in positions of institutional power) that become security actors without narrowing analysis to them. We focus essentially on whose knowledge and practice is deemed authoritative and worthy of adhering to rather than assuming particular actors inherently are.

This also connects us nicely to the approach to audience outlined above, where it was mentioned that securitizing actors will seek to produce "the audience" as *their* audience. In doing so, the speaker also reiterates themselves as one who can speak, is heard, and is adhered to (or can act with authority) just as it produces those who are worth speaking to (and why). Authority and legitimacy in both the subject-position of speaker and what they can say are thus intertwined in the construction of the audience. As other actors reiterate and challenge these constructions, they thus challenge and change the construction of authority. Considering this as part of a securitizing discourse thus allows us to observe how authority interacts with securitizing moves rather than assuming a relationship based on the Copenhagen School's assumptions regarding security.

The Meaning and Logic of Security

Revising these analytical concepts is only half the battle, however. We might be able to recognize multiple audiences, the powerful yet varied role of context, and an expanded number of security actors, but to capture the different claims to security within the US Ebola response, expanding our understanding of security is perhaps most important of all. Indeed, security ultimately lies at the heart of these other problems. It is the emphasis on exceptionalism that leads the Copenhagen School to conceptualize the audience as being just "receptive" and the securitizing actor as the political sovereign. The recognition of security's sedimentation also diminishes the role of context in meaning construction. In altering these other concepts, we implicitly challenge the meaning and logic of security that fuels the Copenhagen School's approach. We must now do so explicitly.

To start with the meaning of security, one popular response—and one in line with the above discussion of context—is to offer a contextualist approach (Ciută 2009; labeled by Neal 2019, 50). Here, the analytical priority is the meaning of security *as constructed by the actors*, not just any definition the analyst brings in. This requires paying attention to how actors employ not only the term *security* but also terms connected to it: *threat*, *danger*, *risk*, and so on. It demands an understanding of the contextual clues that might suggest a linkage to security, such as past threats (equating Ebola to terrorism, for instance) or practices (surveillance or the deployment of the military).

Despite the promise of such an approach, however, there remains one problem to address. It is crucial to analyze the political construction of security, yet it is also equally important not to dismiss the insight of discursive sedimentation. Not all claims to security are effective. Particular articulations carry more weight than others. Wæver (1995, 48–49) is also right to note that certain progressive understandings (in the discipline of international relations, largely) have defined themselves in direct contrast to the national security meaning. While he then problematically uses this to dismiss these alternatives, his premise that the national security approach dictates the discipline's mindset on security remains a poignant one. Consequently, while the basic idea of analyzing security as a political construction remains, it requires a careful application, one attuned to the genealogy of security and the dynamics of power circulating within it.

A promising avenue to address discursive sedimentation while not making it determinative lies in a concept suggested by Huysmans (1998a): the *thick signifier*. This approach observes security as a signifier that receives its meaning from being linked to other signifiers (such as "war" or "protection"). It is thus open to multiple and different discursive formulations, as security is linked to different signifiers. Yet, it is also not *entirely* malleable and open to any and all new linkages. It has "thickness," meaning relationships with other signifiers (such as "war," "enemy," "defense," "the state," and all those associated with national security) that are historically, politically, and/or socially sedimented (Huysmans 1998a, 233). This conceptualization is thus in line with the Copenhagen School's approach to security's meaning, but with a crucial difference: these thick relationships are not *definitive* of security, and the term remains open to alternative contextualized meanings and contestation. Security can therefore be recognized for its sedimentation as the Copenhagen School insists, but this is not then *petrified* into the only meaning of security. Adopting this perspective thus enables a consideration of the multiple ways Ebola was constructed as a security threat without denying the potency of the national security discourse. It promotes analysis that considers how security's thickness posed challenges and opportunities for particular actors as they articulated competing discourses, with some affirming this thick understanding (the representation of Ebola as an external threat to the US, for instance) and others seeking to challenge it (the representation of Ebola as a threat to West Africans). It also permits an examination of just how security is connected to—and receives meaning from—other signifiers, allowing an examination of how context intersects with the construction of security.

While this may address the question of how to conceptualize security's malleable yet sedimented meaning, it does not entirely address the question of how to capture security's logic. This can be problematic, as demonstrated by Claudia Aradau (2004, 2008). For Aradau, claims to security that rely on alternative meanings, particularly progressive ones, are always self-defeating, undermined by the "Schmittian politics at [their] heart" (Aradau 2004, 399). What Aradau is claiming is not that security only has one meaning, but that it adheres to a logic of exceptionalism that—regardless of the meaning ascribed to it—inevitably traps security practice in exclusion, violence, and sovereign control. Aradau's point is important. We must indeed take seriously the logic of exceptionalism thrumming underneath security and how this might lead even the most progressive meanings to exclusionary, Othering, and controlling practices. We should not dismiss the power of this logic as exceptionalism is ultimately core to what makes security distinctive as a concept. Security, as its most basic conceptual level, is premised on the idea that some issues are too urgent, too threatening, and too *exceptional* to be left to normal politics.

Yet we also need to remember the many different ways this can manifest. As the critical security studies literature discussed in the previous section demonstrates, exceptionalism is a far more diverse and contestable site than Schmitt—and the Copenhagen School—consider it to be. It is also a phenomenon located *within*, rather than beyond, politics. It cannot be assumed to take a particular form, despite the Copenhagen School's insistence with the existential threat, elite decisionism, and emergency measures. Nor can it be claimed to always have the exact same effects in rendering politics autonomous, extralegal, militarized, or elitist. The potential for all of this might be there, lying at the heart of the *concept* of the exception, but *practice* is always maneuvered through political interactions. Exceptionalism is thus a political phenomenon; it is potentially transgressive, exclusionary, and violent, but not inevitably so. Capturing this analytically is a challenge, but one worth conquering.

The first step is to recognize exceptionalism as a concept. By this, I mean to acknowledge that exceptionalism is a "conceptual schema," one that highlights key dynamics and weaves them together into an explanation of politics (Doty 2007, 115). In this sense, Schmitt's concept of the exception offers questions of sovereign power, mass identity and the friend/enemy relationship, and the boundaries of permissible/legal action. It presents a "norm" being transgressed, highlighting a sense of political "rupture," but also asks the analyst to define the norm and the transgression. Huysmans (2004, 325–327) has taken this a step further, identifying the core of exceptionalism as the relationship between the rule of law, political leadership, and popular will and what happens to these relationships when the constitutive political principle becomes the fear of violent death. Using exceptionalism as a concept—rather than a blanket description that fits Schmitt's ideal—thus illuminates key dynamics and their potential political relationship and can be used critically to examine ambiguities and contradictions between realities and these conceptual claims (see Doty 2007; Neal 2019, 89).

This brings us to the second, most critical step: the rejection of Schmitt as the conceptual center of exceptionalism and an opening of the concept's key tenets to possibility. This is not to reject Schmitt altogether but to recognize Schmittian exceptionalism as just one potential form of exceptionalism. Exceptionalism is not always "where it is supposed to be" but may manifest in places "away from the centre" (Neal 2010, 149). Exceptionalism is defined by questions of intensity (the real possibility of violent death), transgression (breaking or shifting political limits), and authority (the decision and sovereign power), as well as pointing to the relationship between the people, the sovereign, and law/norms. Yet these questions and relationships can vary dramatically in their manifestation, forming a spectrum of political possibilities for each. At one end, we could observe what Bonnie Honig (2009, xv–vi) terms *de-exceptionalizing the exception*, a shift toward the "ordinary" as a site for exceptionalist politics. The Paris School and the broader literature on risk exemplify this, with their emphasis in dispersed, bureaucratic authority, the temporal elongation of intensification from imminent threat to potential risk, and the tiny transgressions within "normality" (Bigo 2002; Aradau et al. 2008, 149–150; Lund Petersen 2011; Kirk 2020). On the opposite end of the spectrum lies Schmittian exceptionalism, but also the work that criticizes it as inadequate in capturing this more extreme end of security practice, such as Aradau and van Munster's (2011, 112) work on catastrophe. More importantly, however, is what lies in between.

So how do we analyze this, empirically? Essentially, we ask a series of questions: who has "decided," what temporality of danger is proposed, whether legal or political normality has been transgressed, and what all of this might (and does) look like in the specific context in which it has occurred. Does this articulation of danger propose a transgression of current political limits through the sovereign based on an imminent threat from an enemy, as Schmitt suggests? Does it entrench a perception of vulnerability, necessitating smaller alterations from within bureaucratic organizations or even in everyday civilian activities? Or does it lie somewhere in between, and, if so, how are these differing ends reconciled?

Securitization as Process

Before finally bringing these conceptual changes together into a set up of securitization, it is worth finishing on a note about what this means for the basic idea of securitization. By this point, we have left behind the idea of securitization as a speech act, a single moment of elite speech that constructs security. Instead, securitization is a process. It is reiterative and productive, not a single moment of speech but multiple claims that contest and change. It involves the construction of a threat but also the construction of an accepting audience and speaker authority. Context infuses each part but is also reproduced and altered itself in this process. Emergency measures—which can take many different forms with varying levels of exceptionalism—reiterate these constructions but also feed back into this process, becoming new sites for debate. By considering this a reiterative process, we move beyond simply identifying a case of securitization to explore what it actually means and does to claim an issue like the Ebola outbreak as a security threat. We can delve into the precise components of construction without assuming them: what threat(s), what referent object(s), what audience(s), what security actor(s), and what emergency measures? Why did particular constructions dominate and why did others fail to resonate? Did constructions change through interacting with others? And what did this mean for the practical response, within both West Africa and the US? Conceptualizing securitization as a process with these understandings of audience, context, actors, and security provides us the foundation to answer these questions.

The Set Up: A Discursive Approach to Securitization

Wæver suggested that scholars of securitization "set up" their framework, based on the core theory. This chapter has so far done this in long form, outlining the conceptual foundations for an approach to securitization that best captures the multiplicity, contestation, and change within the US response to Ebola. However, before we conclude and move to the application of this set up, let us outline exactly what it looks like and how it translates to analysis.

Ultimately, I use a discursive approach to securitization. A discursive approach to securitization transforms the speech act from a moment of elite construction to a reiterative and productive process, open to multiple voices and meanings and overlapping with contextual discourses in its constant "play of practice" (Milliken 1999, 230). It focuses on how security is constructed, examining how it is articulated through linked representations of threat, referent object, actor, audience, context, practice, and, of course, the meaning and logic of security itself. It thus allows a consideration of how security can be constructed in different ways, either slightly or entirely: the same issue (Ebola) can be linked with different representations of audience, context, threat, referent, and so on. The key is thus the relationship *between* these representations rather than the single linkage to security (Milliken 1999, 229). We can trace these linkages, identify these discourses, and consider just where the key differences lie. A discursive approach to securitization therefore provides a solution to the initial conundrum of this book: how to analyze multiple securitizing discourses.

Just as crucially, it permits an examination of the other puzzles: contestation and change. A discursive approach is *inherently* intersubjective. Some erroneously suggest that discourse focuses exclusively on "text," typically that of elites (and thus the speech act and discourse are equivalent). This is not true. Discourses are not text. Discourses are a series of utterances or, more accurately, the underlying "social, political, and cultural phenomena" or meaning that give these utterances their performative significance (Dunn and Neumann 2016, 2–3). Indeed, in direct contrast to the speech act, the power of discourse lies not in its utterance but in its *iterability*, or its ability to be cited, recited, and changed through such reiteration. Discourses *must* be reiterated. They are unstable systems, requiring "work to 'articulate' and 'rearticulate' their knowledges and identities" (Milliken 1999, 230). The result is a social process: securitizing moves are not merely performed but must be reperformed and dispersed between multiple actors to stabilize and thereby become productive.

It is in this intersubjective production and reproduction that contestation and change exist. As discourses are rearticulated, the representations within can shift in accordance with new events, interaction with other representations, or even purposeful efforts to destabilize or silence the discourse. Indeed, as Doty (1996, 6) describes them, discourses have "an overlapping quality," where their "exterior limits are constituted by other discourses that are themselves also open, inherently unstable, and always in the process of being articulated." We must therefore consider not only how discourses are articulated and rearticulated but how they do so while overlapping with other, potentially competing discourses. There is always, in other words, a "*play of practice*, or *struggles* over which discourse should prevail" and in what precise form (Wilhelmsen 2017, 170).

Drawing together this basic discursive set up with the above discussion of each conceptual component, we can form a series of questions for analysis:

- Which discourses, containing which representations, seem to reach the point of hegemony? How are these challenged, in what ways, and by whom?
- What is the threat being constructed? To whom or what is it threatening?
- Who is the audience for each discourse? Are they the same or different and how do they compete?
- What contextual discourses are drawn on and how?
- Who is speaking and acting? Whose knowledge is important and worth knowing? How is their authority constructed, reiterated, and/or challenged in processes of authorization?
- Is the thick understanding of security reaffirmed or challenged in these articulations? What forms of exceptionalism are invoked and what political effects do they have?
- What emergency measures or security practices are enacted, and which are challenged?

This approach thus considers securitization as a contested political process of discursive construction and reiteration, one that occurs over time and between actors.

Specifically, I employ a poststructuralist understanding of discourse rather than the neo-Marxist-inspired critical discourse analysis used by Stritzel (2011, 2014). This follows in the example of Hansen (2006, 2011),

Wilhelmsen (2017), and Song (2015), ultimately fulfilling a suggestion made by Stritzel (2014, 29–30) to align securitization theory closer with theorists such as Foucault, Derrida, and Butler. I choose this approach for reasons outlined in the discussions on audience and context: it eschews the temptation to find single, objective explanations for securitizing moves and success (which cannot account for difference, change, and contestation) and allows for multiplicity *and* agency. The former is guaranteed through poststructuralism's emphasis on productive power, or how the world is given meaning through discourse (and thus can have multiple, competing meanings). It should be stressed here that, despite some claims, poststructuralism does not assert that there is no "real world." Rather, it focuses on how we can only know this world through our "traditions of interpretation," or discourse (Campbell 1998, 6). The latter is assured through the insistence on discourse as an iterative process, moving beyond elites to consider how actors engage, reiterate, and challenge particular representations. Agents operate within the conditions of possibility circumscribed by discourses and are defined and rendered authoritative (or, conversely, denied authority and legitimacy) through them, yet they are never entirely bound by them. The need for reiteration means that discourses are always open to change by actors, with new discourses also a possibility. The Fearbola counterdiscourse, which resulted from numerous commentators challenging the prominent securitizing discourses, is a clear example of this.

Yet the question of agency also draws out important critiques from competing strands of securitization, particularly by those who blame the undertheorization of the audience on Wæver's poststructuralist influences. It is important not to lose sight of these critiques. The focus on discourse can—and has—lead to a lack of attention to audiences as well as other actors who are silenced or disempowered within the discursive space (see Hansen 2000; Bertrand 2018). We must ensure that the questions of "who can(not) speak" and "for whom is action undertaken" remain central. In addition, it is important not to lose sight of the power dynamics, institutions, and resource struggles that entwine with and are reproduced by discourses, as highlighted by approaches such as critical discourse analysis.[1] Discourses are part of a *dispositif*, alongside "institutions, architectural forms, regulatory decisions, laws, administrative measures, scientific statements, philosophical, moral, and philanthropic propositions" (Foucault 1980, 194), as outlined by other Foucauldian approaches. We must consider how processes of authorization connect to institutional power structures, for instance. How is President Obama's authority recognized, challenged, or qualified? Which experts (and forms of knowledge) are deemed authoritative and which are not? How does this connect to institutional arrangements? And it is important to be clear about the role of practice, often seen as ignored or diminished by poststructuralist approaches (Hameiri and Jones 2015, 49). With this latter concern, we must reiterate that practices are not merely the by-products or effects of discourse. They are *part* of discourses—a different medium to the linguistic and the visual but still a form of representation and meaning production that carries the discourse (Hansen 2006, 20; Aradau et al. 2014). Quarantines and airport screening, for example, produced as much meaning as textual claims that health workers returning from West Africa were dangerous. Ultimately, this discursive approach to securitization has benefited from an engagement with other approaches. It is heavily poststructuralist, but an approach that critically synthesizes insights from the wider securitization literature.

In translating this theoretical framework broadly into method, what results is a critical reading of texts. Such a method involves identifying how the chosen issue (the Ebola outbreak in West Africa) is represented as threatening: in what ways, by what actors, to which referent objects? At first, this is akin to content analysis, in the sense of identifying just how Ebola and the outbreak were depicted. Using NVivo, I manually coded these depictions according to their representation of threat: economic threat, the threat of mutation, the threat of global circulation, the threat of a US outbreak, the threat to West African state stability, the threat to West African lives, the threat of fear, and the threat to "you." This was an inductive and reiterative process. As new common representations became apparent during reading, I reread earlier texts to observe where and when they first appeared.

Yet discourses are systems of signification, where meaning is produced through the relationships between these signs (Milliken 1999, 229). I thus moved beyond this initial identification of representations to trace how they were linked and differentiated and how they were linked and differentiated to other representations such as audience, authority of security actors, context (historical, social, and political), meaning of security, exception, practice, and, ultimately, competing discourses. Again, I manually coded these representations and then focused on the linkages and differentiations between them that provided meaning to the whole. Representations outlining the threat of a US outbreak, for instance, commonly appeared alongside representations of the US audience as fearful, West Africans as dirty, diseased, and a source of threat, President Obama as abdicating his role of sovereign, government experts as political agents, and a travel ban as common sense. It is important to remember that these did not always appear together in one single text. Rather, the linkages between these various representations were common enough across the many texts analyzed that they formed a system that produced meaning: a discourse. In essence, securitization theory and its key concepts (as revised above) provide a neat initial framework to map securitizing discourses, pointing to the key representations to be observed. Yet it is also important to not be limited to these concepts and be open to the possibility of other representations.

In the chapters that follow, we can observe how this basic method takes two complementary forms. The first, in "The Basic Securitizing Discourses," focuses on mapping the basic securitizing discourses and identifying the key representations and their linkages/differentiations. In identifying and analyzing these representations, I focus on the textual mechanisms of presupposition, predication, and subject-positioning (see Doty 1993, 1996; Shepherd 2021, 34–35). Presupposition refers to the creation of "background knowledge that is taken to be true" (Doty 1996, 10). Analytically, the focus lies on observing how statements will "presume access to commonly shared structures of knowledge" (Dunn and Neumann 2016, 110). This is common in references to context. Claims that West Africa did not have the "expertise" to combat Ebola, that its populations adhered to "myths" and "superstitions," and that its governments were corrupt were often articulated with little to no evidence. However, they did not need evidence to be understandable for the US audience. They relied on a contextual narrative of Africa as the Dark Continent: dirty, diseased, incapable, and threatening. Predication focuses on how predicates ("describing words") are linked to the subject (Shepherd 2021, 34). Subject-positioning, meanwhile, points to the relationships between subjects, which may be that of "opposition, identity, similarity, and complementarity" (Doty 1993, 306). These two mechanisms are often intertwined. Predicates surrounding West Africa, for instance, often constructed a juxtaposition to the US: "they're almost bereft of health care facilities, of anything close to what we would consider to be reasonable" (John Isakson, in CHELP 2014, 39). "They" (West Africa) were "bereft of health care facilities," a point given full meaning by the reference to US as "reasonable."

The following chapter, "Securitizing Ebola," then moves from this deconstructive focus to examine the *play of practice*, specifically how discourses manifest, interact, and change in real-world practice. Structuring this analysis through Hansen's (2006, 28) concept of key events, it focuses on where, how, and by whom these representations (and their linkages/ differentiations) were articulated, rearticulated, challenged, and changed. Here, I focus the analysis on how these events were variously represented, how these representations operated within the larger securitizing discourses, how these representations—and discourses—clashed over these events, and how this process altered both these discourses and the conditions of possibility within which the US response occurred. Importantly, I employ Julia Kristeva's (1980, 66) concept of *intertextuality* here. Intertextuality is premised on the recognition that all texts "make references, explicitly or implicitly, to previous ones, and in doing so they both establish their own reading and become mediations on the meaning and status of others" (Hansen 2006, 49). In this case, I use this idea to examine how actors reproduced competing representations, with some managing to do so in a way that rendered the original representation invalid. This chapter thus positions the previous chapter's analysis (outlining the multiple ways Ebola was securitized) within the actual process of securitization itself.

Conclusion

The fundamental goal of this chapter was to set up the book's analysis of the US response to Ebola. As outlined in the introduction, this response is widely—and aptly—noted as a case of securitization, where an issue is constructed as a security threat. Indeed, securitization theory is a remarkably valuable approach. It not only highlights this construction but offers deep insight into the politics of security, namely the intersubjectivity of this construction, the sedimented national security meaning, and the logic of exceptionalism with all its potential benefits and worrying detriments. It is thus an approach to keep and well worth using to analyze the US response.

Applying securitization theory, however, is easier said than done. The founding Copenhagen School may have given us an insightful theory and a parsimonious and intuitive framework, but there are also a number of gaps and limitations within this approach. The theory does not merely recognize security's sedimentation, it petrifies it into the single, only meaning of security. The logic of exceptionalism remains rigidly bound to the ideal of Carl Schmitt, missing that the bulk of contemporary security practice does not sit within these extremes. The audience is undertheorized, undermining the claim to an *intersubjective* construction of security. The role of context is also lacking in detail. Securitizing actors seem to be limited to political elites, another byproduct of the Schmittian confines of the theory. Each of these is a problem in and of itself, but together they problematize our efforts to analyze the multiplicity, contestation, and change evident within the US response to Ebola.

These are, of course, not new critiques. They have animated an enormous body of second-generation securitization literature. This same body of work has also provided multiple answers to these gaps and limitations, including numerous schools, models, strands, or alternative approaches to securitization. Rather than simply adopting one of these approaches—which would ignore their cross-fertilization, the diversity within each broadly defined camp, and the value and limitations of each—this chapter focused on how this literature has answered each of the core limitations. Tracing the explanations and answers provided, it ultimately came to see the value in a poststructuralist discursive approach to securitization. A discursive approach allows us to consider the role of the audience, the significance of context, multiple actors beyond political elites, the changeable and contested meaning of security, and the wide variety of exceptional practices and forms of politics that it might engender. It views these attributes as constructions within an inherently intersubjective process, where competing securitizing discourses overlap with, clash with, and change one another. Tracing these discourses, their interaction, and their changes over time and between actors will thus allow us to view the process of securitization as it occurred in the US during the Ebola outbreak.

Ultimately, this follows Wæver's suggestion to use securitization as an "idea theory," one in need of "set up" when used empirically. Indeed, it should be reiterated that the goal here was not to produce an alternative model or school of securitization. It was simply to consider how we might use securitization to answer the questions I ask of the US Ebola response: how was the outbreak securitized, in what way, to what effect, and how do we explain the contestation and multiplicity evident in this case? In this vein, it follows the path well-trod by second- (and perhaps even third-) generation securitization scholars: it takes the Copenhagen School's insightful, innovative, but parsimonious idea theory of securitization and considers how best to employ it to understand the messy complexity of security politics. And it is to that messy complexity that we now turn.

3 The Basic Securitizing Discourses

Introduction

Having set up the analysis in the previous chapter, we can now turn to the analysis itself. Here, we return to the puzzle outlined in the introduction: the securitization of Ebola within the US domestic context and the multiple, competing claims to security that characterized it. This research is thus animated by two questions: Why and how was the Ebola outbreak in West Africa securitized in the US? How was this securitization of Ebola contested and what did this mean for the US response to the outbreak? Answering these questions is a task that contains two steps: first, identifying and mapping the multiple securitizing discourses that were evident and, second, considering how these discourses interacted within a broader process of securitization.

This chapter is devoted to the first step. Here, I outline the basic securitizing discourses that were evident during this process, identifying the threats, referent objects, securitizing actors, audiences, emergency measures and, crucially, understandings of security they produce. To do this, I adopt Hansen's (2006) idea of *basic discourses*. Basic discourses are analytical ideal types; they are "stylised representations of what a phenomenon would look like when its internal logic is fully maximised," aimed not at capturing the nuances of articulation but the broad strokes of a discursive field (Dunn and Neumann 2016, 106). Yet my outline of basic discourses differs from Hansen's in one crucial respect. While she emphasizes identity as the central "nodal point," my conceptual focus on securitization places an additional requirement. The aim, after all, is not to identify any and all discourses concerning the Ebola outbreak but to focus primarily on the debate surrounding its construction as a security concern. In the vernacular of discourse analysis, I am effectively coming into my analysis with a preset "nodal point," "the so-called quilting point or point de capiton around which the shifting of signifiers is temporally halted and meaning installed" (Edkins 2002, 72). By this, I mean that security serves as a crucial center to these discursive structures, a "partial fixation" that is used to order other signs but is empty on its own, only provided meaning through these linkages (Laclau and Mouffe [1985] 2014, 98–99). I am thus not merely mapping the basic discourses, but the basic *securitizing* discourses that can be observed within the wider securitization of Ebola.

To do this entails detaching these discourses from one another and considering them separately. Yet the production and (re)iteration of these discourses did not occur separately; the signifiers used, the connections made, and the meanings proposed built on one another and changed in accordance with continued interaction. Splitting the discourses from this interaction is therefore inherently partial and risks eliding points of commonality and overlap. Yet there is a benefit to this. Focusing first on the basic securitizing discourses allows a detailed examination of how each "system of signification" functions internally and seeks to create a coherent and unified "regime of truth." It also "identif[ies] the main convectors of discussion" between them (Hansen 2006, 84). In other words, exploring these discourses as self-contained systems might overstate their independence at the risk of obscuring their intertextuality, but doing so allows me to demarcate their differences, their internal logic, and their attempts to produce a regime of truth that could be fixed over others. The result of this is an illumination of the debate's boundaries: the threats observed, the audiences spoken to, the authorities to be listened to, and the measures that needed to be implemented or rejected. The second step—the next chapter—then explores the space in between these boundaries, where these broad regimes of truth met, clashed, aligned, and altered one another.

Specifically, this analysis (as outlined in the previous chapter) involves first identifying the common representations of Ebola as threat, including the kind of threat, its source, and the threatened referent object. It then involves tracing the linkages between these representations and other key securitizing representations (audience, authoritative actors, emergency measures, security, etc.) and differentiations against others. Part of this is identifying frequently appearing phrases or descriptors (similar to a content analysis). Another, more prominent component of this analysis is examining the presuppositions, predicates, and subject-positioning within these texts and around the subject of Ebola. This is ultimately an interpretive form of analysis, conducted through close and repeated readings of the gathered data.

From this analysis, we can observe three basic securitizing discourses. Each of these offered a distinct referent object, conception of the outbreak's threat, proposal for appropriate measures undertaken by authoritative actors, and justification within an approving audience, and each was grounded within an understanding of security's meaning and exceptionalist logic, together forming a "regime of truth" for the outbreak and the US response. I have labeled each of these three by their distinctive emphases: Potential Global Catastrophe, America Under Threat, and Helpless West Africa. Yet there is also a fourth discourse we must consider here, one that is not securitizing but still crucial to this process of securitization: the Fearbola counterdiscourse. I consider it a counterdiscourse as it operated solely to challenge these securitizing discourses yet was not explicitly desecuritizing.

The Potential Global Catastrophe Discourse

The Potential Global Catastrophe (PGC) discourse is the first we consider here for one simple reason: it was the official discourse, the meaning provided to the Ebola outbreak and US response to it by the Obama administration. Within this discourse, in other words, are not only representations of Ebola's threat, but also justifications for President Obama's response, including representation of the president, the US federal government, and their vision for American security and foreign policy. The primary securitizing actors here are thus President Obama and his administration (including government agencies such as the CDC) but also the politicians and segments of the media that reiterated, defended, and/or expanded on the Obama administration's depiction of the outbreak and response.

The PGC discourse is labeled for its three most distinctive representations: the referent object, the threat, and the temporality of these representations. Within the PGC discourse, the referent object is *global stability* and the US's vulnerability within it. The threat is *catastrophic damage*, or damage that could either irreversibly alter the current system or be unacceptably excessive in its cost to it. Finally, each of these are viewed through the temporal prism of *potentiality*, not *immediacy*. Yet while this set of key representations covers the crux of this discourse, it is only the surface of a more complex process of sign linkage and differentiation, one equally reliant on constructions of the audience, authority, and knowledge. To map this discourse thus requires examining this process.

The key representation lying at the heart of the PGC discourse is that of Ebola and the outbreak as a "threat to regional and global security." This phrase appeared in two of President Obama's (2014b, 2014e) speeches in September 2014. Yet, on its own, such labeling is generic. It tells us little about just how Obama and those who reiterated this framing understood Ebola's *securityness*. One thing that is notable just from this phrase, however, is that the threat is to *regional* and *global* security rather than *national* or *human* security. To understand further, we look to Obama's (2014b) elaborations on this identified threat:

> And if the outbreak is not stopped now, we could be looking at hundreds of thousands of people infected, with profound political and economic and security implications for all of us. So this is an epidemic that is not just a threat to regional security—it's a potential threat to global security if these countries break down, if their economies break down, if people panic. That has profound effects on all of us, even if we are not directly contracting the disease.

The "regional security" threat is thus the "hundreds of thousands of people infected," a threat given clearer meaning in another September speech: "in Liberia, in Guinea, in Sierra Leone, public health systems have collapsed [, e]conomic growth is slowing dramatically [and] . . . this disease could cause a humanitarian catastrophe across the region" (Obama 2014e). As both speeches emphasize, however, "regional crises can quickly become global threats" (Obama 2014e). The global security threat is thus given meaning through the linkages with state breakdown, economic collapse, and societal panic.

The referent object here is thus the US yet also not the US: it is the implications for "us" that are threatening, but these implications are temporally and spatially distant, detached, and deferred rather than direct. The threat is not the immediate danger of Ebola but the future and possible effects of the outbreak ("if these countries break down, if their economies break down, if people panic"). Spatially, the direct threat is to global stability—the political, economic, and security status quo—with the threat to US national security arising from its positioning within "a world as interconnected as ours" (Obama 2014f). Yet we can observe here presupposition: Obama does not explicitly outline the "profound effects on all of us" that these regional problems will have, but assumes his audience understands the linkage via background knowledge. This background knowledge, of course, is the dominant conceptualization of disease as a national security threat outlined in the introduction, where the state (the US, in this case) is threatened through the capacity for outbreaks to threaten their interests and capacity to act and function.

Obama's speeches provide a good introduction to the PGC discourse and its key representation of Ebola's threat. Focusing on Obama's speeches also reveals that the PGC discourse was the official discourse, or that of the Obama administration's response. Yet discourses are not constituted solely by a couple of texts. Obama's speeches did not form the PGC discourse on their own. If we look to the statements, interviews, conferences, and documents of the Obama administration, other politicians, and parts of the media (including news reporting and political commentary), we see this basic representation reiterated. Importantly, this basic representation of Ebola as a threat to global stability is expanded in this reiteration. It moves beyond the presupposition to outline the linkages between the regional crisis and global security—economic instability, state breakdown, and the global circulation of Ebola—and links to other key securitizing representations such as the audience, actor authority, emergency measures, and the exception.

The amount of expansion, however, differed between these threats. Expansions of the economic instability representation were least common and more frequently appeared within the media than in the statements of other members of the Obama administration or other politicians. It did, however, appear in all of the media examined, spanning both the ideological remit (Fox News to MSNBC) and genre (reporting and commentary). Some reporting highlighted the economic costs for the region (Nossiter 2014c, 2014f; Sengupta 2014; Sengupta et al. 2014). Others, however, explicitly noted the wider implications of the outbreak for the "international economy" (Juan Williams, in SRBB 2014e; Daniel Lucy, in Newsroom 2014g), where the outbreak would cause enormous "costs" or "disruption" for "us" (Foege et al. 2014; Kristof 2014a, 2014b; Pollack 2014b). Addressing the outbreak was thus good economics, while a lack of appropriate early action was a "shortsightedness" that would "never [be] tolerate[d] . . . in private behavior" (Kristof 2014b).

Another form of this economic linkage was to depict the outbreak as a disruption to an otherwise positive narrative of "Africa rising," where Africa (as a whole) was portrayed as a rising (future) economic power (Gerson 2014a; Mui 2014). The outbreak thus potentially ruined the "opportunities" for the US in "the world's last major economic frontier" (NYT 2014a). It is worth noting that this economic threat was frequently articulated in conjunction with the other two main threats outlined within the PGC discourse: state breakdown and the global circulation of the virus (see Foege et al. 2014; SRBB 2014e; Newsroom 2014g). Indeed, it was rarely outlined as a threat on its own and instead placed within the list of worries commentators had regarding Ebola's global impacts. Accordingly, while greater details of the threat were given, it remained within Obama's framing of the outbreak's threat as a broader, multidimensional one to global stability.

The representation of Ebola as a threat to West African state stability was slightly more common. Notably, it was particularly common in the statements of Obama administration officials and members of government agencies. Here, the outbreak was represented as a politically destabilizing force, one that risked undermining "the social fabric of entire communities" (Foege et al. 2014; Candy Crowley, in SOTU 2014a) within the "fledgling democracies" of West Africa (Ariel Pablos-Méndez, in CFA 2014a, 22; see also Josh Earnest, in White House 2014b; Liptak 2014). Again, this was framed less as threatening in terms of its impacts on *these* states and more in relation to the possible impacts on *American* security and political interests, as outlined by the State Department's Bisa Williams to the first congressional hearing on Ebola:

> We do not want the virus to erode the capacity of African countries to address other important national and regional challenges. We want to ensure these countries remain strong, strategic allies to the United States in a region facing serious development and security challenges. (CFA 2014a, 30)

Unlike the representation of economic threat, which tended to remain general, this threat of state breakdown was often constructed in more specific forms. The possibilities were rife: "regional war" (Kent Brantly, in CFA 2014b, 57), where the collapse of the state would unleash the "post-civil war conflicts" that simmered under the surface of states such as Sierra Leone (Karen Bass, in CFA 2014b, 9; see also John Berman, Early Start 2014b; Cooper 2014); the "nearby" terrorist groups such as Boko Haram taking advantage of an Ebola-facilitated power vacuum (Garrett 2014b);

an "uptick in refugees trying to escape across borders" (Siakor and Bowier 2014); and even the prospect of terrorist groups using Ebola as a biological weapon (Noack 2014). Interestingly, the few West African voices that were able to break into American media and speak in their own words (rather than being interviewed and quoted) also often highlighted this prospect, pairing their cry for aid with a reminder to act "before the entire region collapses into chaos" (Siakor and Bowier 2014; see also Cooper 2014).

Underpinning this construction of threat was a representation of (West) Africa itself as fragile or incapable. The state was "battered by political dysfunction and civil war" (McNeil 2014b) and "almost dysfunctional" (Anthony Fauci, in AC360 2014b; see also Garrett 2014a), with "health system[s that have] largely collapsed" (Onishi 2014a). The people were variously described as "rock-hurling mob[s]," "angry," "superstitious," and "ignorant" (Callimachi 2014; Daigal 2014; Jones 2014; McCoy 2014e, 2014e; Paye-Layleh 2014; Schmemann 2014a). These predicates combined with a clear subject-positioning of the inferior West African Other against the modern and capable US, with one Republican senator (John Isakson) evidencing his belief that West Africa was unable to contain the outbreak by referring to them as "almost bereft of health care facilities, of anything close to what we would consider to be reasonable" (CHELP 2014, 39). Such depictions were especially prominent within the media and were not limited to specific media sources or forms (television or print). This is important to note, as these depictions of West Africa frequently served as the context or background for reporting or commentating on the crisis. In doing so, they effectively acted as the presupposition, the taken-for-granted understanding of West Africa.

As will be explored later, this West African Fragility representation was common to all the securitizing discourses. Yet it resulted in different meanings depending on the linkages that were made. When linked to the construction of possible state breakdown in West Africa, it served as the context for that threat. The Ebola outbreak was thus a match to the powder keg of these unstable states, who had barely rebuilt themselves after grueling years of civil war and violence. This representation may seem to contradict the "Africa rising" narrative, but together the two constitute (West) Africa's temporal identity within the PGC discourse. (West) Africa may be a source of future economic opportunity and political partnership, but it continues to face "challenges" that always keep this rise on the cusp of disintegrating

(Susan Rice, in Today 2014b; WP 2014b). Moreover, it justified the US as the security actor. Indeed, since West Africa's "backwardness" was the cause of the outbreak, then America's modernity—"the kinds of capabilities that only America has" (Obama 2014b)—would end it.

The third and final of the main constructions of threat within the PGC discourse is one of Ebola's threat to global circulation, or that Ebola would spread beyond its natural "containment" in (West) Africa. This was a biopolitical representation of the disease's threat. Ebola was understood as contained to Africa, but the outbreak threatened to alter the disease's global circulation (or lack thereof), becoming "unmanaged." Media commentators and experts worried specifically about Ebola reaching countries with "underfinanced and overwhelmed" public health systems, such as India (NYT 2014d), and then "periodically travel[ing] to America" (Kristof 2014c). Again, the US was the deferred referent object here, as CDC Director Frieden (in FNS 2014a) repeatedly made clear: "the single most important thing we can do to protect Americans is to stop the spread of disease around the world."

A particularly important variant of this construction of the threat was that of mutation, or the threat of the virus becoming *biologically* unmanageable:

> If we don't make that effort now, and this spreads not just through Africa, but other parts of the world, there's the prospect then that the virus mutates, it becomes more easily transmittable, and then it could be a serious danger to the United States. (Obama, in MTP 2014b)

Notably articulated by Obama (in MTP 2014b) in early September, reiterated by various reporters and commentators across the media landscape (see, for instance, Gerson 2014c; Klein 2014; Liptak 2014), and also—and perhaps most crucially—outlined by Michael Osterholm (2014b) in a widely requoted *NYT* opinion piece, the prospect of mutation was one of the most common of the explicit constructions of threat. Like the West African Fragility representation, the threat of mutation appeared in other discourses, notably the America Under Threat discourse. Indeed, as Obama's quote above suggests (with the mention of becoming a threat to the United States), there was considerable space for overlap between the two on this point (which did occur in practice, see next chapter). Yet again, the precise linkages differed, with this representation employed in slightly different ways. Obama, members of his administration, public health officials (such as Fauci and Frieden), and the various reporters and commentators who reiterated the PGC discourse typically framed the threat of mutation as an amplification of the global spread concern. If Ebola spread for too long, it could mutate into a different form. And while Ebola's current form was dangerous, it was *known*. Officials and experts frequently assured reporters and—by extension—the audience that "we know how it works" (Christensen 2014; see also Tom Frieden, in CFA 2014a, 9; FNS 2014a; Obama 2014f; 2014h). Mutation, particularly the possibility of an alteration in its virulence or mode of transmission, threatened this knowledge and thus the ability to manage the virus.

Underpinning these threats—though the above in particular—was a particular form of knowledge production. As mentioned previously, the threat was temporally and spatially deferred: a future economic shock, the disintegration of currently intact states, and the alteration of Ebola's circulation to beyond its contained geographical zone or its biological form beyond what was known and manageable. Yet this temporal focus did not just change *when* the outbreak was threatening but also *what* precisely was threatening about it. The threat was not the outbreak as it currently stood but what it *could* be: it was the "prospect" of mutation (Obama, in MTP 2014b), or the "risk" of Ebola becoming endemic in West Africa (Kristof 2014c). Moreover, this was not simply a mention of plausible trouble but the possibility of complete *catastrophe*. Ebola did not simply risk economic turbulence, state fragility, or a few cases throughout the world but could potentially massively disrupt growth, cause complete state collapse, turn West Africa into a hotbed of war and terrorism, and spark a global pandemic. Yet there was a crucially grounded element to this: these were possible future scenarios *if the current situation continued*. Speakers outlined these potential threats in relation to what was already occurring, such as uncontrolled spread within West Africa leading to global circulation (for instance, Van Susteren and Serrie, in Greta 2014a). Speculation was always premised on what was known and calculated, not what was unknown and imagined. This was thus speculation from certainty, and speakers sought to draw boundaries and emphasize this position of certainty, especially as opposing approaches moved to the uncertain.

This conjectural knowledge basis was also crucial in understanding the exception constructed by the PGC discourse. On the one hand, the outbreak was represented as exceptional in terms of its potentially catastrophic effects. Obama's (2014b, 2014d, 2014e) speeches in mid-September are illustrative here, describing the outbreak as "an epidemic of the likes that we have not seen before" as it was "spiraling out of control" and "spreading faster and exponentially." It was an urgent ("we have to act fast") and extreme ("we have to move with force") threat that thus required "a major increase in our response": the deployment of the US military (Obama 2014b). Reporters, commentators, and other politicians of both parties observed this announcement as appropriately exceptional, with one commentator describing it as a "dramatic escalation" that indicated that the Obama administration was serious about the security threat posed by the outbreak (Chris Matthews, in Hardball 2014a). Attempts to stabilize this representation even drew on other "known" exceptions such as terrorism and ISIS. Such representations, especially in the earlier parts of the response, crossed party lines. Republican Sen. Lamar Alexander (in SRBB 2014d), for instance, remarked to Fox News: "We need to give it the same sort of urgent response that we give to the terrorists in the Islamic State, and we need to do it while we can, while we can still control it."

On the other hand, however, speakers also suggested that the deferred and uncertain threat qualified this exception. The military was deployed, but under the framing of it as a uniquely humanitarian actor: "our armed forces are essentially the biggest NGO on the planet for helping people" (Charles Krauthammer, in SRBB 2014e). Obama (2014f) equally stressed that it was due to the military's capacity for "logistics" and "engineering"—"and . . . our Armed Services are better at that than any organization on Earth"— that soldiers were being deployed. This was not explicitly framed as a "war on Ebola." More significantly, extreme forms of exceptionalism—forms of decisionism and significant disruption to legal and regulatory norms—were explicitly denied. A clear example of this is the Obama administration's refusal to enact travel and trade restrictions, as justified by CDC Director Frieden (in FNS 2014a):

> You know, we are dependent and we are part of the world. There are 50 million travelers from around the world that come to the U.S. each year that are essential to our economy, to our families, to our communities. We're not going to hermetically seal this country.

The exception, in other words, did not extend so far. It did not extend into the US itself nor demand such a dramatic disruption of the norm. Instead, the Obama administration constructed an exception that questioned and stretched the limits of a solely public health response while refusing to transgress them entirely. A "more appropriate" form of emergency measure was offered in the form of enhanced airport screenings, where particular bodies (West Africans) were subjected to greater and more intrusive surveillance. While this might constitute an excess to civil limits, it was framed by the Obama administration instead as a stricter (enhanced) enforcement of a legal norm (Jeh Johnson, in CDC 2014b; see also Josh Earnest, in White House 2014c). In this vein, airport screenings were an exercise of state power that both adhered to the sense of exceptional action yet also sought to mitigate its excesses and keep it within the normal legal framework.

A similar perspective was taken on drug development. All of the securitizing discourses—and indeed, representations of Ebola more generally—included representations of pharmaceuticals as potential Magic Bullets for the outbreak. A treatment provided to two infected health workers in August garnered an enormous amount of media attention as a "secret serum" that might cure the disease (see, for example, Brooke Baldwin, in Newsroom 2014c; Savannah Guthrie, in Today 2014b; Pollack 2014a). While the White House (2014a) and Obama (2014a) himself insisted that such a cure would not come in time (or was needed) to halt the outbreak, they still devoted extra funding to this research and, crucially, loosened some of the restrictions around testing and use such as through compassionate use of experimental medications and Fast Track or "animal rule" approval (Largent 2016). Yet again, all of these were exceptional actions *within the norm*. This was not a breaking of FDA rules so much as a stretching of them. This is ultimately a logic of *risk as exception*, rather than the Schmittian extreme. It sought management of the danger, folding the exception back into the norm rather than completely disrupting or overturning it.

Authority also remained dispersed, rather than the centralized decisionist sovereign expected of the Schmittian exception. The only move that suggested a centralization of power was the designation of Ron Klain as the Ebola response coordinator, colloquially known as the Ebola Czar, on October 17. The framing of this act is crucial, however. Obama and the White House depicted Klain's controversial appointment not as a single sovereign to decide and control the response, but to act as "an implementation expert" with "extensive management experience" (Josh Earnest, in White House 2014d). Obama remained the ultimate authority, the sovereign to whom Klain answered, but even Obama's authority was rarely represented as absolute. He did not decide alone; his decisions—and White

House policy—were frequently depicted as only following well-publicized consultations with public health officials. Indeed, his political authority was premised on this: he listened to those who "knew," and he acted "based on the science, based on the facts, based on experience" they offered (Obama 2014i).

Obama's authority as president was thus intertwined with the simultaneous construction of his public health officials—namely Frieden and the CDC—as the experts or expert authorities. Again, all the media sources analyzed reiterated this construction, though they did so to varying degrees and at different times (see next chapter). What is key for the PGC discourse is not only the reiteration of this representation, but the use of this to authorize the other PGC representations, including President Obama's political authority. See, for instance, this reporting from Marc Siegel on Fox News's Hannity (2014a):

> He told me, Dr. Frieden, that they are going to use the same kind of quarantine that they use for SARS, which is actually spread through the air. This is much, much harder to get. And Dr. Fauci, the head of the National Institute of Allergy and Infectious Diseases, the most prominent infectious disease expert in the country, and I have a big interview airing from him tomorrow, he told me that it's an infinitesimally small chance that [returning health workers] would spread it.

Fauci—"the most prominent infectious disease expert in the country"—was reiterating the PGC representation of risk to the US (the "infinitesimally small chance"). In reproducing Fauci's position as an expert authority, this representation is not only reiterated but strengthened. With regards to Obama's political authority, this linkage to expert authority served well at points during the response and public debate, but it became a crucial weakness in the later stages of the securitization process, as the next chapter will explore.

Also key to performing this subject-position of political authority was connecting to a particular representation of the audience. For Obama (2014i) to speak and act on behalf of the American people, he needed to identify exactly who or what they were:

> America in the end is not defined by fear. That's not who we are. America is defined by possibility. And when we see a problem and we see a challenge, then we fix it. We don't just react based on our fears. We react based on facts and judgment and making smart decisions.

The audience—the American people—was rational, guided by science, and compassionate. Notable here is *who* was most frequently making this claim. Members of the Obama administration and experts more commonly uttered these representations than members of the media, who tended to represent the audience as more fearful and even irrational. Indeed, many of these audience representations were offered in response to these competing claims to justify the representations above and the practices they enabled as being in line with the "real" American people and their values. In bringing back two health care workers (Kent Brantly and Nancy Writebol) to the US for treatment in August, Frieden (in FNS 2014a) responded to the "lot of fear" evident "from all the social media sites" by asserting: "I hope and I'm confident that our fears are not going to overwhelm our compassion. We care for our own. We bring people home if they need to come home."

The three subject-positions are ultimately inextricable: "we"—Obama, his experts, and the American people—are rational and compassionate actors, premising decisions on "the science" (which was solid, certain, and held no gaps or disagreements). They were thus automatically aligned on the nature of the threat and the most appropriate response to it. Ultimately, underpinning this nexus of agent/audience representations was one of America as a whole: the Indispensable Nation. This is a long-running contextual discourse in American foreign policy. Commonly attributed to former secretary of state Madeleine Albright, the "indispensable nation" was described by Albright as "stand[ing] tall and . . . see[ing] further than other countries into the future" (USDoS 1998). In essence, the term presupposes the idea that only the US has the capacity and benevolence to assure global security. Accordingly, when members of the Obama administration—including President Obama (2014c), Secretary of State Kerry (2014), and National Security Advisor Susan Rice (2014)—explicitly and consciously reiterated this representation in their statements on the Ebola response, it was a clear effort to ground and contextualize their understanding of the crisis (and best response) in a powerful image of the American Self.

The PGC discourse, ultimately, formed an intersection of traditional forms of security and risk to produce an exceptionalism that merged components of both. The regime of truth primarily articulated by President Obama and his administration was a discursive combination that allowed for the amplification of threat while restraining the response to the establishment of (an American) normality in West Africa. Yet this left it tenuous, a balancing act between the extreme and the mundane. Obama's opponents—both his direct Republican opposition and those otherwise favorable to him—took full advantage of this, using the glimpse at the exception to proclaim that Obama did not go far enough.

The America Under Threat Discourse

Perhaps the main competing discourse to the official discourse of the PGC was what I have labeled the America Under Threat (AUT) discourse. The AUT discourse shares commonalities with the PGC discourse, particularly some key representations (the West African Fragility representation, for instance) but also has a distinctly different approach to the thick signifier at its heart: security. There is some level of overlap between the two here: both could be described as vaguely "national security" discourses of disease, reproduced and recontextualized to the Ebola outbreak. Yet there are some crucial differences in how they reproduced this national security understanding, which resulted in distinct—and competing—securitizing discourses. Unlike the PGC discourse, which merged risk and security logics to construct the outbreak as a potential threat to global stability, the AUT discourse ultimately articulated the pure Schmittian ideal, the idea of protecting the (American) Self against the (West African) Other and permitting decisionist sovereign power to ensure it. Yet it did so also by focusing on hypothetical scenarios, again blending notions of risk but in a way that still produced an imminent and existential threat. It did so through securitizing the outbreak as a possible *direct* threat to the American people.

Being the main competing discourse to the official discourse (that produced by the Obama administration), it should come as little surprise that the main securitizing actors most commonly iterating and reiterating the AUT discourse were Republicans and conservative media commentators, especially in the latter stages of the response. However, just as the PGC discourse was reiterated by some of these figures, the AUT discourse also was not limited to these actors. Media reporting from all media sources (including the more Democrat-aligned MSNBC/NBC) reiterated key representations that formed the AUT discourse. Some Democrats too repeated these claims of danger, exception, and emergency measures. Accordingly, we should note the primacy of Republicans and conservative media in forming this discourse, particularly as their position outside of and in opposition to the government influenced both their representations and their capacity to speak and be heard, but we should not consider the AUT discourse as *solely* a Republican/conservative one. This again demonstrates the value in examining discourse: it moves away from assuming particular actors only engaged with one discourse to examine the specific regime of truth and consider just how powerful it is in setting the conditions of possibility.

At the heart of the AUT discourse was the construction of the American people as the referent object to the "threat" of Ebola. This construction occurred through two forms. The first was through a construction of the collective Self, where the threat was to "us." In essence, this was representation through subject-positioning, where the speaker and the audience were positioned as one (Americans). This was most common within media reporting and commentary, particularly the television news broadcasts. The fears, desires, and interpretations of the speakers were considered as those of the audience (and vice versa), whether this equivalence was accurate or not. Occasionally, this was explicit, as speakers articulated what they assumed to be the audience's response: "If I'm in that hospital or around that hospital, I think I'd be very, very nervous" (Eric Bolling, in The Five 2014b). Others offered their own reactions as indicative of audience response: "that sent a chill through my spine" (Bill O'Reilly, in TOF 2014b). In making this equivalence between the speaker and the audience, this representation not only centered the American referent object (who was, in this case, literally the person speaking/reporting/commentating on events) but also sought to reiterate that the fears regarding Ebola were rational and understandable.

The second form of representation constructed the referent object through claiming to speak on behalf of it. This might seem similar to the aforementioned construction of the Self, but it differed in the sense that it was a construction of authority rather than one of shared victimhood. Politicians frequently reiterated this particular representation, namely through representing themselves as the sovereign protectors their people—the audience—clamored for. New Jersey governor Chris Christie (in FNS 2014c), for instance, positioned himself as simply fulfilling his democratically provided mandate "to protect the safety and health of our citizens." We can observe two forms of subject-positioning here, both in Christie's representation of himself as the protector and in his implied representation of "our citizens" as requiring this protection and thus the referent object. While this subject-positioning was particularly prominent within the statements of politicians, media figures also laid claim to a form of authority (as knowledge providers) through asking the questions their audiences ostensibly

wanted answered. This was particularly common in televised news reporting (rather than commentary), where news anchors and interviews justified
their questions as being those that the audience ostensibly had: "Obviously,
there are a lot of people in the United States concerned about the spread
of this disease, this disease spreading to anyone else" (Anderson Cooper, in
AC360 2014b).

While focused on the referent object, the nature of authority was equally
central to the AUT discourse. Opposing politicians—as well as media commentators who defended their actions or challenged Obama's—claimed
that the definition of political authority was to protect the people from
any and all external risks they faced. As Sen. Ted Cruz (2014a) argued, West
Africa might be suffering more right now, but the president's job demanded
that he prioritize the risk to the American people first:

> We need to do everything we can to contain this outbreak, to help the people
> who are suffering in Africa and to prevent this epidemic from spreading. But our
> first priority must be to protect the health and safety of American citizens. The
> Constitution sets forth the federal government's responsibility to "provide for the
> common defense." That should be the president's focus.

This is important for two reasons. Firstly, it rejects a simplistic and inac-
curate assertion that AUT proponents entirely disregarded what was occurring in West Africa or that they uniformly believed West Africans to be
not worth helping. While some figures may have held this perspective, the
majority saw this as an issue of prioritization rather than complete dismissal. Secondly, but related, it illuminates the moral underpinning of
this discourse. This was, ultimately, a claim to the meaning and purpose
of security. At the heart of the AUT discourse and its prioritization of the
American referent was a claim to security as being fundamentally about the
protection of the Self (and "our" people). The loss of life in West Africa was
thus a "tragedy," one worth acting to mitigate, but not the "obligation" or
"responsibility" that security imbues authority with (Cruz 2014a; Dennis
Prager, in Hannity 2014a; Bill O'Reilly, in TOF 2014b). Indeed, in the earlier
stages of the response, this led some conservative commentators on Fox
News's talk shows to suggest that Ebola was *not* a security issue, particularly when compared to "real" security concerns such as terrorism (The Five
2014a; SRBB 2014d).

As this suggests, the precise construction of the threat was enormously
important for the AUT discourse. It was not enough to simply insist a threat

exists to the audience. The threat had to be fixed as a direct and existential danger (the "real possibility of violent death"), one that justifies the moral prioritization. Accordingly, of the three securitizing discourses, the AUT discourse is perhaps the one that is most focused on the disease itself. Speakers frequently focused on its mortality rate, its disturbing symptoms (for instance, "horrific internal and external bleeding," Erin Burnett, in EB:O 2014a), its transmission through bodily fluids, and its potential for mutation. Reporters covered "Ebola scares" in the US with a reminder to their audiences that the disease "can kill up to 90 percent of those it infects" (Erin Burnett, in EB:O 2014e) and the effects are so rapid that "you can be fine in the morning and dead by dinner time" (Brian Williams, in Nightly News 2014a). Some notable articles—including one that was requoted in the *Washington Post* (McCoy 2014a)—even positioned these attributes toward the reader/viewer, emphasizing the effects Ebola could have on "you":

> Your own immune system, now completely out of control, attacks every organ in your body. Tiny blood vessels burst everywhere and you begin slowly to bleed to death. The whites of your eyes turn red, your vomit and diarrhoea are now charged with blood and large blood blisters develop under your skin. (Gatherer 2014)

By decontextualizing these depictions—moving away from the West Africans actually suffering from these effects—the emphasis becomes the dreaded disease of Ebola, with the American referent object implied through the focus on "you." Moreover, such depictions—especially in television news reporting—were also frequently paired with questions regarding the risk of spread to the US homeland, reiterating the construction of the referent object, and linking it to the horrible experience of Ebola.

Ebola itself was thus the threat and this was represented as a self-evident, internal quality, which justified the level of fear "the audience" ostensibly felt in relation to it. Again, however, this simplicity masks the more complex process of construction involved. Three intertwined constructions became integral to this: the contextual discourse of pandemics and the role of intertextuality in connecting Ebola to this, the production of knowledge through imaginaries and hypotheticals, and the grounding of these in a long-running contextual discourse of (West) Africa as the Dark Continent.

The threat of Ebola, as some commentators noted, was one reminiscent of other infectious diseases. Ebola was connected to HIV/AIDS, influenza (and specific variants such as H5N1 and H1N1), and SARS, with this linkage used to draw meaning from these "known" diseases to provide meaning to the Ebola outbreak. In some cases, this was to give the specific threat of muta-tion clearer significance by equating it to the ease of transmitting influenza (Osterholm 2014b). Others, meanwhile, sought to remind the audience that "national security threats come not only from malevolent countries or groups" (WP 2014c). Here, Ebola became the potential pandemic:

> Could we have a worldwide pandemic? The Spanish flu in 1918 killed 21 million people, the plague in the 14th century killed 25 million people; I'm not saying that's going to happen, I don't know what's going to happen. (Rand Paul, in Boyle 2014)

This was a reiteration of a contextual discourse, one Priscilla Wald (2008) has termed the *outbreak narrative*. At its core, this discourse suggests that the world is "due" for a devastating pandemic, one where an "emerging or re-emerging infectious disease" (whether natural or weaponized) spreads across the globe via contemporary globalization processes and causes mas-sive loss of life, economic collapse, and drastic societal change. Crucially, this narrative erases the specifics (including the socioeconomic factors) of an outbreak's origins, spread, and response. In linking to this discourse, the Ebola outbreak was subsumed into this generic story.

Of course, this outbreak narrative was apparent within the PGC dis-course as well. Yet, as with other basic contextual representations that overlapped between these discourses—such as the West African Fragility representation and the Indispensable Nation representation—this basic idea took different forms depending on how actors linked it to the other key representations within the securitizing discourse. Within the PGC dis-course, it was linked to the representations of the US as the *deferred* refer-ent object and the threats of economic shock, global circulation, and state breakdown. The Obama administration, reporters, and commentators thus reproduced the outbreak narrative to focus on global vulnerability and the wider implications for global stability, whereas the AUT discourse, with its referent object as the American people and the threat of Ebola, reproduced the outbreak narrative with a specific focus on the massive loss of life it entailed. To restate this more simply, the PGC reproduction of the outbreak narrative did so to emphasize the risk to the world, while the AUT discourse reconstructed it to emphasize the existential threat to *us*: "given modern air travel and the latency time of the disease, the virus will jump borders and threaten lives . . . even here in the United States" (Rep. Chris Smith, in CFA 2014a, 1).

Intertextuality was vital in this reconstruction. Media figures frequently drew on fictionalized accounts of disease outbreaks—namely those already based on Ebola, such as Richard Preston's 1994 book *The Hot Zone* and the 1995 film *Outbreak*—to provide specific illustrations of the potentiality of Ebola (see, for instance, Cohen 2014; Fareed Zakaria GPS 2014; Osterholm 2014b). Yet, in line with the outbreak narrative, the generic story was just as vital. Republican Congressman Blake Farenthold (in CHS 2014, 51), for instance, explained that he was "skeptical" of the CDC's Dr. Toby Merlin's assurance that Ebola was not a domestic threat as "every outbreak novel or zombie movie you see starts with somebody from the Government sitting in front of a panel like this saying there is nothing to worry about." Accordingly, speakers and their audience did not need to know or refer to the specifics of the outbreak in West Africa; they simply drew on the stories from pop culture—in which Americans were typically central—to (re)produce these threat constructions.

Underwriting these claims was a production of knowledge through conjecture. The outbreak as it was currently known was not the threat for the AUT discourse. Rather, the threat lay in a possible future scenario where it traveled to the US. This made the AUT discourse similar to the PGC approach in terms of stretching the temporality and certainty of the threat. In contrast to the PGC approach, however, which saw the president, members of his administration, and figures in the media speculate from what was currently known and certain, the speculation within the AUT discourse was premised on a foundation of *uncertainty*. The claim was not simply that the future threat was uncertain, but that the *current* situation could not be entirely certain. It could not be known or quantified. Ebola was unknown. There was "so much mystery surrounding this illness" (Anderson Cooper, in AC360 2014b), including the way it was transmitted ("my suspicion is that it's a lot more transmissible than that," Sen. Rand Paul, quoted in Kaplan 2014a). To insist otherwise—that Ebola was known and that we could rely on this knowledge—was thus to provide "a false sense of security" (Rep. Tim Murphy, in CEC 2014b, 187).

Accordingly, the future threat was not merely speculated, but *imagined*. Rather than "what might happen," the AUT discourse relied on "what ifs":

I recently visited with the leadership of one of Texas's largest health care systems about their precautions to counter Ebola. I asked how many Ebola patients they could reasonably handle with these protocols. "Six or so," they responded. What if, God forbid, we saw 8,000, as in West Africa? They had no answer. We shouldn't risk finding out what that answer might be. (Cruz 2014a)

Republican Sen. Rand Paul (quoted in Killough 2014) also asked his audience to "imagine" a terrifying scenario: "if a whole ship full of our soldiers catch Ebola." General John F. Kelly (quoted in Garamone 2014) also weaved a tale of "ifs" in outlining his worries of Ebola "com[ing] to the Western Hemisphere . . . particularly Haiti and Central America," where the threat was "mass migration" of these imagined infected immigrants. All these cases rely on a foundation of uncertainty for their speculation. They focus on what "we don't know we don't know" (Rep. Bill Johnson, in CEC 2014a: 144–145) and argue that the US needed to base their response on this hypothetical future as it was the only way to protect the American people. A common phrase here—and one that became especially common for Republican politicians—was "an abundance of caution." Since the threat could not be completely known, every possible form it could take needed to be considered equally.

The final, but perhaps most integral, representation of Ebola's threat was that of race and geography. Like the PGC discourse, the AUT discourse's construction of threat was firmly linked to the representation of Ebola as an African disease, where the outbreak was a direct result of West African Fragility. Similar constructions of the people as "ignorant," "backward," and "violent" were offered, as were those surrounding the ineptitude of the states' political, economic, and social systems. It is again worth noting that these depictions tended to be far more common in the media than the statements of politicians, even those who more closely adhered to the AUT discourse.

However, the temporal construction of this "fragility" differed. Unlike the PGC discourse, where (West) Africa was ultimately capable of "evolution," the AUT discourse constructed (West) African fragility (and even failure) as a perpetual, inherent, and insurmountable attribute of the region and its people. Africa (not just West Africa) had "customs" and "superstitions" that meant they could never control such an outbreak (Greg Gutfeld, in The Five 2014a). The "infrastructure" and "mistrust . . . in these countries" was "so profound" that "experts around the world" ostensibly believed spread was likely (Christine Romans, in Early Start 2014a). It was similarly "curse[d]" by corruption (Dennis Prager, in Hannity 2014a). These predicates were used as though they were *innate*: not simply the result of "falling behind," but a marker of what was intrinsically African. This was, in essence, a reconstruction of the Dark Continent discourse, a long-running contextual discourse of Africa as a place uniformly rife with war, poverty, and disease.

Ultimately, when linked to representations of Ebola's "deadly" nature, the American referent object, and the uncertainty of knowledge, the representation of West African Fragility transformed the threat into one of contamination. (West) Africa was a petri dish of disease, and its people the receptacles that moved it over borders: "There's about 200,000 Africans from countries hosting the deadly Ebola virus who hold temporary visas to the United States" (Andrea Tantaros, in The Five 2014a). Even those who did not live in West Africa were not spared from blame: an article from *Newsweek* even suggested that West African immigrants to the US were "smuggling" Ebola into the US through their "cultural touchstone" or "ethnic delicacy" of "bushmeat" (Flynn and Scutti 2014). West Africans themselves became sources of threat.

It should thus be little surprise that AUT proponents strongly advocated for practices of containment. If the threat was from "outside" agents, the response necessitated a denial of entry to the "inside." Two practices were proposed to do this: a travel ban and quarantines. The former was premised on a strict geographical division: the denial of physical entry to the US homeland. Indeed, this was described by most proponents as "closing our borders" to West Africa, creating an ostensibly impenetrable fortress to the infection. Republican politicians particularly advocated for this practice, with a significant number releasing statements during the month of October to this effect (Cruz 2014a, 2014b; Topaz 2014). Justifications for this practice reiterated the key representations of threat and referent within the AUT discourse. Sen. Ted Cruz (2014a; quoted in Kaplan 2014), one of its strongest proponents, described it as a "common sense" and "prudent" way to eliminate "the risk": containing the West African bodies understood to contain it. In contrast, the (PGC-related) prospect of simply screening West Africans via a rudimental physical examination and questioning—and thus permitting them some level of agency to decide their own threat—was "truly insane" (Bill O'Reilly, in TOF 2014b; see also Blake Farenthold, in CEC 2014b, 51).

Quarantines retained this idea of physical separation but did so by creating spaces of exception "inside" the US. In contrast to the travel ban, quarantines were focused solely on American citizens, mainly returning health workers and reporters. Unlike West Africans, they had a "right" to return home and be treated through the US health systems should they be infected, but their "choice" to enter the Dark Continent rendered them a threat and permitted a limitation on those rights:

> Even though there's a dispute over the details of [the quarantine], there is now a national consensus, as there should be, that if you return from that zone, particularly if you have a fever, you can be in quarantine; which of course is an infringement on your civil liberties. [But] we seem all to agree that quarantine—meaning the state depriving you of liberty—is the way to go in a potential epidemic. (Charles Krauthammer, in SRBB 2014g)

Like the travel ban, this was a proposal to eliminate risk through controlling risky bodies. Controlling these (white, American) bodies was more contentious, however, and necessitated a greater degree of justification. Those politicians who implemented such measures—notably the governor of New Jersey, Chris Christie, and the governor of New York, Andrew Cuomo—thus paired their claims to the exceptional nature of the threat with a representation of people as untrustworthy. One could not "count on a voluntary system" (or "honor system") of self-monitoring, "when you're dealing with something as serious as this" (Gov. Chris Christie, in FNS 2014c).

Both of these practices were ultimately claims to the Schmittian exception. For AUT advocates, the extraordinary nature of the threat meant that the sovereign needed to decide who entered and who did not, who held rights and whose could be denied, and whose bodies could be watched, removed, or enacted on. This was especially apparent in the way that the PGC discourse's "enhanced" airport screenings were reproduced by these commentators and politicians. They were "a complete smoke and mirror approach to the virus" (Dennis Ross, quoted in Marcos 2014), "defie[d] logic" (Bobby Jindal, in Topaz 2014), or simply an exercise in "politics" that would "risk entire populations" (Kelly 2014). Travel bans and quarantines, in contrast, were frequently depicted by these political opponents as "common sense" (Christie, in FNS 2014c; Cruz 2014a, 2014b; Scott Brown, in CNN 2014a). They filled these apparent gaps in the screenings: they eliminated the risk entirely through denying any and all bodies that might pose it and they relegated these bodies to the control of the US state, refusing duplicitous or malicious actors the agency to cause harm.

Containment was not the only exceptionalist practice demanded by AUT proponents, however. As mentioned in the discussion of the PGC discourse, all the securitizing discourses represented pharmaceuticals as a Magic Bullet to stop the virus. Yet, like the other shared representations, the linkage of this basic representation with those distinctive to the AUT discourse resulted in differing meanings. Specifically, in relation to the "extraordinary circumstance" that was the (apparent) threat of Ebola to the US, it was deemed necessary to "break every fail-safe that exists at the FDA" (Richard Burr, in CHELP 2014, 66). This demand frequently appeared in the congressional hearings around Ebola, as members of Congress asked panels of government experts why more of these Magic Bullets were not available. Even safety concerns—maintained by the Obama administration—should not slow down the process:

> **Borio:** But there are situations where if the risk is believed to outweigh the benefits based on the available science we—it is called a clinical hold. We basically tell the sponsor that the study cannot proceed in volunteers at this moment until some adjustments are made and the benefit-risk profile is more favorable.

> **Burgess:** There is a broad understanding at the Food and Drug Administration that this is no ordinary time, correct? (CFA 2014a, 74)

The "extraordinary circumstance" of Ebola meant that extreme transgressions were not only justifiable but required.

At its core, the AUT discourse centered on the Schmittian exception. Premised on the moral foundation that "security" was about "our" protection, actors (predominantly, but not exclusively, Republicans and conservative media) produced a threat to the Self/audience that was the possibility of violent death rendered real: the disturbing disease from Africa. They thus demanded the sovereign to act accordingly: to decide, to centralize and unify authority, to control, to break rules and norms, and to focus attentions first and foremost on "us," the people. Yet this discourse also challenged the Schmittian narrative. While the threat was understood as existential, it was not imminent. It lay within a hypothetical future, one based on conjecture and uncertainties (or the construction of uncertainty) that proposed questions that "we shouldn't risk finding out" the answer to (Cruz 2014a). This enabled the exception to stretch further and justify the denial of liberties and a disruption to the response even when proponents recognized there was no current threat. This made this discourse particularly powerful within the broader debate, especially against the official PGC discourse, its restrained form of exceptionalism, and its deferred threat and referent object.

The Helpless West Africa Discourse

The final of the three securitizing discourses is what I label the Helpless West Africa (HWA) discourse. Like the AUT discourse, it is named primarily for the referent object it constructed: West Africans. The HWA discourse shares commonalities with the PGC and AUT discourses, notably overlapping in key representations such as West African Fragility, the US as the Indispensable Nation, and the Magic Bullet of pharmaceuticals. Yet it differs from these two discourses fundamentally at its core, the thick signifier: security. Rather than a reproduction of the national security discourse of disease, the HWA discourse could instead be described as a *human security* approach to the outbreak.

Human security discourses, as explored in the introduction, emphasize security from the perspective of those fundamentally insecure: not so much those who face sudden disruptions to their freedoms but those who are perpetually without them. To identify the HWA discourse as one of human security is therefore to identify it as one making a claim to security based on who was *most* insecure:

> There are two realities about the current Ebola epidemic in West Africa—one from inside the infected zone, and another from outside of it. . . . The clash of these two realities is to be expected, given the extreme circumstances. It is like this when one disadvantaged corner of the world is beset by a calamity, and the rest of the world peers in, anxiously and imperfectly, from a vantage point in which no one is worried about relative order, a constant supply of electricity and running water, and air-conditioning. (Nossiter 2014c)

The people of West Africa were insecure not merely in the sense of facing an outbreak but also in a more pervasive sense of being vulnerable to the very worst and most immediate outcomes. In essence, the HWA discourse was seeking to securitize *for* West Africa in the American context, asserting that the direct, immediate, and *real* security threat ("fear" and "want" in its many guises) to be that faced by West Africans. As the quote above from Adam Nossiter's reporting highlights, some even constructed this referent object by challenging claims to others, namely the US: "the real tragedy and epidemic that is going on is not in the United States. It's in Africa" (Powers, in SRBB 2014b).

The HWA discourse is a discourse that was articulated, rearticulated, expanded, and defended from actors across the media and political land-scape rather than the general (but imperfect) partisan divide that might be drawn between the PGC and AUT discourses. However, the media was the primary site for this discourse, with newspaper reporting and commen-tary specifically more common in reiterating these representations. *Outside* commentators—academics, global health experts, and members of non-governmental organizations such as Samaritan's Purse and Médecins Sans Frontières—were also notable proponents of this position. Importantly, actors who otherwise tended to align with other discourses, including President Obama, also occasionally reiterated this discourse. While there is already evidence in this chapter of actors shifting in their perspectives and moving between discursive positions, the HWA discourse and its key rep-resentations saw this more often. News anchors, for instance, occasionally disrupted *their own* speculation of the threat to the US with "but the situa-tion in West Africa is horrific" (Anderson Cooper, in AC360 2014a). Obama (2014b, 2014d, 2014e), Secretary of State Kerry (2014), and other govern-ment officials (see Higginbottom 2014) constructed their claims of excep-tionalism by meshing their fears of potential global catastrophe with the recognition that the current and immediate threat was in West Africa. This might seem to diminish the HWA discourse's role as a contained regime of truth, but—as the next chapter will demonstrate—it actually attests to the power of the HWA discourse in setting boundaries for the public debate even if it did not dominate it. Its construction of threat, referent object, audience, identity, and exception are thus important to understand.

At the heart of the HWA discourse are two representations of threat and referent. The threat of Ebola was the "perfect storm" of poverty, underde-velopment, corruption, and neglect that both led to the outbreak and made its consequences worse (Piot 2014; quoted in Achenbach and Dennis 2014). It was not simply a sudden and singular problem but was tied irrevoca-bly with the wider dimensions of West African insecurity. We can observe here, again, the West African Fragility representation. Health systems were "already fragile" and "overburdened" (Johnson 2014), with "the very basic public health protections and practices simply [not] exist[ing]" (Ezra Klein, in All In 2014a). This was variously due to their recent emergence from civil wars (Chris Smith, in CFA 2014a, 3) and the "decades of poor political decision making, bad investments, and brain drain" by governments, leaving them with zero capacity to protect or serve their populations (Johnson 2014). Again, however, meaning was produced through the linkages between these representations and that of Ebola's threat. West African Fragility was not concerning because it left the affected states vulnerable to collapse but because it meant there was an "absence of effective care" and thus "many are dying needlessly" (Kim and Farmer 2014). The outbreak was thus not "the triumph of an unstoppable disease" but "a failure of economic and human development" (Ezra Klein, in All In 2014a).

This construction of threat centered on a claim to certainty and immediacy. In clear contrast to the PGC and AUT discourses, the HWA approach constructed a threat image of the outbreak as it *currently* was. USAID's Stephen O'Connell (2014) even described the emphasis within some media reporting on the potential threats as a worrisome and potentially destructive focus on "alternative views of the future" based on "caricature[s of] the present." This is not to claim, however, that these speakers did not consider any potential or long-term effects. Deputy secretary of state, Heather Higginbottom (2014), told the US Senate Committee on Appropriations that she was highly concerned with the broader effects of the outbreak on West African insecurity:

> Beyond the epidemic's immediate effects, fewer children are being vaccinated against other communicable diseases, an increasing number of people lack adequate food, and economies have been severely impacted. In short, the Ebola epidemic is not only a health crisis—it is a global threat.

These articulations, however, were still grounded in a claim to certainty and immediacy, albeit one that was based on a comparison to the other discourses.

This representation of the Perfect Storm was thoroughly intertwined with the second key representation of the HWA discourse: the Helpless West African referent object. As mentioned, the HWA discourse's most fundamental difference from the other two securitizing discourses was its emphasis on the West African referent object. In some cases, commentators depicted this referent object with agency and respect, even when acknowledging the need to help (Benton and Dionne 2014; Breen 2014; Seay and Dionne 2014). More commonly, however, this was another reiteration of West Africans as the inferior Other, emphasizing the suspicion, ignorance, and occasional violence of locals and the inadequacy and corruption of governments. Yet there was a crucial difference here. These depictions of the West African Other connected to predicates of *passivity*:

> There's no way to describe the scenes from West Africa other than just heart-wrenching, gut-wrenching. And the images of a pregnant woman being turned away from a hospital on the—and she's on the verge of collapse, or of men and women dying on the streets, their children orphaned, and a lot of hopeful nations working to plant the seeds of prosperity and open societies now suddenly battling a brutal epidemic. (Kerry 2014)

The West African population was not made up of agents to be blamed but helpless victims to the overwhelming structures of poverty and government inadequacy.

Part of this is the question of what is depicted (pregnant women collapsing, men and women dying, and children being orphaned) and what is not (the West Africans that made up the bulk of the health workers, for instance). Another is how it is depicted. Gendered representations were particularly prominent in news reporting that constructed this passive West African. Women's—particularly mothers'—agony was highlighted (see Fink 2014d), as was the dead and dying female body, with one long-form newspaper article starting with this "hook":

> Tom Frieden remembers the young woman with the beautiful hair, dyed a rusty gold and braided meticulously, elaborately, perhaps by someone who loved her very much. She was lying facedown, half off the mattress. She had been dead for hours, and flies had found the bare flesh of her legs. (Sun et al. 2014)

As this suggests, the woman herself was rarely the focus. Rather, it was the disgust and tragedy centered on her body and the impacts this had on others. Similarly, children's bodies and suffering were frequently described to invoke helplessness in its most extreme (Fink 2014e; Gettleman 2014; Onishi 2014b). Children, as Helen Berents (2019, 149) writes, are widely idealized as "touchstones of moral purity," where "their suffering can only be read as a failure of the adults that surround them." Alongside women, markers of both pity (the mother's anguish) and disgust (the decaying beauty), they become representations of both sides of West African inferiority: its helplessness and need for protection as well as its ignorance and backwardness.

Ultimately, these constructions of the referent object and the threat produced a moral prescription for action. The Helpless West African, powerless against the direct threat of Ebola and vulnerable to greater dangers, needed salvation. They could not manage it themselves, and thus required the American hero to save them from the abyss. This was a "moral obligation" that America's supremacy burdened them with (Chris Thompson, in CHS 2014, 6; see also Chris Matthews, in Hardball 2014a). Some, moreover, had already answered the call. A key figure within the HWA discourse was the Heroic Health Worker, an individual who had courageously left behind their comfortable and safe existence to save the unfortunate Other. They not only "put . . . their own lives on the line," but did so "for strangers" (Al Roker and Natalie Morales, in Today 2014b). Of course, this was a heroic *American* health worker. The heroism of local health workers was rarely explored, with some notable exceptions in the work of Adam Nossiter (2014d, 2014e; Nossiter and Solomon 2014) from the *New York Times*. For the most part, however, those interviewed were foreign, largely American, health workers (Fink 2014a, 2014b, 2014c; Watson 2014). This was both a continued erasure of West African agency and a reiteration of the inherent righteousness of American action. This was another reiteration of the Indispensable Nation discourse observed previously but also a crucial twist on it. It was represented less as a burden, demanded because of the US's capabilities, and more as a marker of the inherent benevolence of the American people. In other words, it was directly linked to *the audience*: the Heroic Health Worker was offered as a representative of the audience, embodying their values and challenging them to live up to the ideal.

In terms of practice, proponents of the HWA discourse were often in alignment with the PGC discourse, notably the sending of the US military and expansion of funding. Médecins Sans Frontières's president Joanne Liu (2014), for instance, even called for military involvement prior to Obama's (2014b) September 16 announcement and welcomed the decision when made. As one opinion piece in the *Washington Post* noted, while the "militarization of aid" was normally concerning, "th[is] situation is dire" (Dionne et al. 2014; see also Deloffre 2014). The representation of pharmaceuticals as Magic Bullets and the need for loosened restrictions was also evident here. Again, however, the linkage to the other representations altered the meaning. August, for instance, saw a debate rage around the question of who could and should receive experimental treatments, a debate sparked by criticism that the *real* victims—West Africans—were being left to suffer while "all of the stops get pulled out" for "two white Americans" (Erin Burnett, in EB:O 2014e). Yet, in conjunction with the broader understanding of security that lay at the heart of the HWA discourse, some also offered broader prescriptions. The representation of Ebola's threat as a Perfect Storm, or inextricable from the fundamental insecurities faced by West Africans on a daily basis, meant that truly responding to the crisis involved a more comprehensive engagement with (human) insecurity in its many forms. As then-president of the World Bank, Jim Yong Kim, and renowned global health professor Paul Farmer argued in the *Washington Post*, the crisis was ultimately the consequence of these "long-standing and growing inequalities of access to basic health care" (Kim and Farmer 2014). The answer, therefore, was to do something about it, even if this answer would need to wait for the end of the immediate outbreak.

This was ultimately a carefully constructed cosmopolitan formulation of exceptionalism. It was suggested that West Africa faced an imminent, existential threat, yet our common humanity provided a moral prerogative for "us" to act on it. The HWA discourse, in other words, kept the Self/ Other dynamic but rejected the Schmittian identification of this as "friend/ enemy." Instead, the representation of the Other was used to draw them into the "friend" category. They might be in an inferior and lesser position to the American Self, but they were worthy of protection from the threat of Ebola. Accordingly, the exception that they faced demanded immediate and wide-ranging action, beyond what we would "normally" be willing to commit to.

There was also a crucial spatial component to this production of exceptionalism. The outbreak constituted an exception due to its imminence, its capacity for catastrophic destruction, and the moral prerogative that was attributed to the referent object, but this was all firmly situated *in West Africa*, not the US. The exception was spatially contained. Norms and rules could be broken there, but these ruptures were not acceptable within the US. Quarantining health workers (and thus denying their civil liberties), for instance, was not justifiable and even a "violation of human rights" (Kaci Hickox, in SOTU 2014c). One reporter on CNN even openly criticized this practice as deterring American health professionals from volunteering in West Africa, thus making the outbreak worse (Elizabeth Cohen, in TSR 2014e). In this case, the nature of the exception (there) demanded the protection of normal politics (here). A *Washington Post* (2014d) editorial even proposed that the Obama administration and/or the CDC step in more forcefully to assert this "normal" state, even if it meant breaking the norms surrounding the separation of authority (quarantines were part of the state's authority over its public health policy) for the sake of the *real* exception: the threat to West Africa.

Ultimately, the HWA discourse challenged the traditional realist discourse of security (the "thickness" of the signifier) and sought to reproduce the logic of exceptionalism to more cosmopolitan ends, a normative framing that led it to contention with the PGC discourse even when they were aligned at other points. This meaning and logic of security were all constructed through linkage of key securitizing representations—the threat (the Perfect Storm), the referent object (the passive West African), the audience (benevolent), and the most appropriate response (immediate use of the military and long-term building capacity in West Africa)—and differentiation against other representations, namely the American referent object within the AUT discourse. Again, however, nuance and contestation still occurred, namely in relation to the precise nature of West African fragility. Considering the HWA discourse broadly, we can observe a tendency toward the Othered representation of West Africans. Yet some articulations did recognize and problematize this Othering while still insisting on the need to aid West Africa in their fight against the outbreak (Benton and Dionne 2014; Breen 2014; Seay and Dionne 2014). This variation is important to recognize, not only to be thorough, but also because it attests to the broad and unstable boundaries of these discourses. One might reiterate key representations—and thus this regime of truth—while challenging others. The next chapter will explore this in more detail.

The Fearbola Counterdiscourse

So far, this chapter has discussed discourses that aimed to securitize the Ebola outbreak, with contestation limited to what kind of security threat the outbreak constituted and to whom. These three discourses are important to the overarching questions of how Ebola was securitized and why contestation was so rife, but to leave the discussion here would be to miss an equally important counterpoint, one that engaged with each discourse—whether to bolster or destabilize them—in crucial ways. For some media commentators, entertainers, and even a few politicians, the public debate quickly shifted from a rational consideration of the outbreak and how to respond to it, becoming instead "the Great Ebola Freak Out" (Drezner 2014b), suffering not from Ebola but Fearbola (Petrow 2014; Robbins 2014). While they ascribed different causes and reasons to this, this central idea—that the securitized response was one premised on an excess of fear rather than any genuine threat—served as a crucial counterdiscourse to the three securitizing approaches and the AUT discourse in particular.

It is perhaps important to be clear here: I do not consider the Fearbola discourse one of desecuritization. There are two reasons for this. Firstly, Fearbola was largely a discourse about the other discourses. It did not give a solid, stable meaning to the outbreak itself, but rather to the larger debate—the process of securitization—that surrounded it. It cast a critical light on the underlying politics of fear and questioned its operationalization and its racialized and temporal manifestations. In this vein, it fits closer with Judith Shklar's (1998) "liberalism of fear" and Michael C. Williams's (2011) use of this concept in the "securitization of fear" than it does with desecuritization. Secondly, but building from this, it was often employed by advocates of other securitizing discourses. In particular, proponents of the PGC and HWA discourses, especially those within the media, frequently adopted the Fearbola discourse to challenge the AUT framing as it came to prominence in October and November. There was significant overlap between texts (statements/quotes/articles) that were coded for their articulation of the "real" threat to West Africa and those labeling the public response as "hysterical" (see, for instance, Charles Krauthammer, in SRBB 2014b). The Fearbola discourse was thus one of broad strokes, more about the nature of American political discourse than the outbreak itself. Accordingly, rather than going to the level of detail provided above, I will cover the four key representations the Fearbola discourse offered to challenge Ebola's securitization.

The first of these centers on the audience. Claims of Fearbola ultimately represented the audience as somewhat irrational, easily manipulated, and self-centered but capable of greater rational thought. The people were always, by nature, at risk of succumbing to a "primal" (Besser 2014; Farhi 2014) or "millenarian" (Drezner 2014b) dread, a solipsist anxiety of one's own violent death that overwhelmed reason, undermined social trust, and threatened communal bonds. This, moreover, was brought into action not by objective dangers, but through "vivid imaginations, . . . ignorance and natural human fear of the unknown" (USA Today 2014a). Ebola, with "all the hallmarks of a scary disease," easily invoked this atavistic fear (Peter Sandman, quoted in Farhi 2014). Moreover, the audience has been "fed" an "infectious disease narrative . . . for years" through "books and movies about the 'Bug or Virus That Will Kill Us All'" (Smith 2014). It was thus understandable, and perhaps inevitable, for this "primal fear" to run wild. This is essentially a recognition of securitization in the abstract: the encounter with the "passage to the limit"—the real possibility of violent death—that alters the basis for political action and shifts it toward extremity, enmity, and exceptionalism. The Fearbola discourse thus illuminated the politics of fear that operated at the heart of securitization, demonstrating what Shklar (1998) terms the "fear of fear" in liberal politics.

From this recognition of the politics of fear, it was argued, space could be opened for change and contestation. The audience did not have to be defined via its worst tendencies. Greater rational thought was possible.

> America in the end is not defined by fear. That's not who we are. America is defined by possibility. And when we see a problem and we see a challenge, then we fix it. We don't just react based on our fears. We react based on facts and judgment and making smart decisions. (Obama 2014i)

These are reiterations of the Indispensable Nation representation, reproduced to contest the audience representation proposed by the AUT discourse (from, respectively, the PGC and HWA positions). It positions the AUT discourse as a limited view of the American Self, one that is occasionally valid but can be surpassed, and presents its own perspective as this more complete version. Importantly, these constructions do not deny that the audience is irrational, easily manipulated, or self-centered. Instead, they utilize the Fearbola discourse to suggest that the American people can be *more* than their primal fears and move beyond solipsism to "fix problems."

Yet the audience was only half of this equation. The second key representation of the Fearbola discourse shifts this focus to those in the practice of informing: the securitizing actor. Here, the politicians and media commentators articulating the securitizing discourses discussed above were represented as "scare-mongering" (Benton and Dionne 2014; Drezner 2014a) or simply exploiting this primal fear for their own gain. This became particularly prominent as the midterm elections neared in October and November, with this context portrayed by political commentators as a key facilitating factor, if not cause, for the rising fear within these months (Bump 2014b; Jim Acosta, in TSR 2014f; Wickham 2014a). The ire was particularly strong regarding politicians. They were "sleazily glomming onto all this panic in order to score political points," and "reaching for whatever stick lies handy," even if "fantastical and malicious" (Marcotte 2014; Gerson 2014b). These representations of self-serving, opportunistic, or panicked politicians were also portrayed as reasons as to disregard their claims to danger. For instance, Kaci Hickox (in MTP 2014d), a nurse at the center of a public debate over quarantine practices (see next chapter), dismissed the insistence that her quarantine was due to "an abundance of caution" as "really an abundance of politics."

It was not only politicians that were blamed here. The media was also criticized for its fearmongering, even by other media commentators themselves (Gerson 2014d; Marcus 2014; Shepard Smith in SSR 2014). Cable news received the bulk of this criticism (see Marcotte 2014). At the core of such criticism was an idealized representation of the media, which intertwined with that of the audience as easily manipulated with a tendency to irrationality. The media was supposed to be the informed and rational actor, differentiated against the uninformed and fear-driven subject of the audience. This subject-positioning brought with it a moral responsibility: the job of reporters, news anchors, editors, and commentators was to inform and guide the audience toward a more rational and well-grounded understanding of events. For those speaking out against media fearmongering, their colleagues had absconded from this duty, they were not "serving the public" but "disserving it" (Marcus 2014).

The third representation highlighted and directly challenged the common framing of West Africa. Each of the three securitizing discourses relied on a representation of (West) Africa as inferior, backward, and ignorant, though they proposed differing angles and degrees. Those articulating the Fearbola discourse illuminated this tendency. Many focused on the racial component, revealing the prominence of the Dark Continent representation and its particular contextual appeal (and implications) within the US. This was "a long tradition of treating Africa as a dirty, diseased place" (Seay and Dionne 2014). Some highlighted anecdotal evidence that these racialized constructions had detrimental implications for African immigrants and

African Americans within the US (Sanburn 2014) while others took on the subject-position of the West African to highlight its very personal effects (Kidjo 2014). It is here that those who otherwise rearticulated the HWA discourse but contested its depiction of West Africans can be observed. Adia Benton and Kim Yi Dionne (2014), for instance, reiterated that the outbreak required immediate attention and resources, but challenged what they saw as a common trend to "place . . . Africans in two categories: hapless victims and contagious threats." Instead of "waiting for Western aid," they argued, we should provide equipment and training to the "capable" and "knowledge[able]" West Africans "who would do most of the work." Such critical interventions were rare but spoke to the capacity to represent the outbreak differently without losing sight of its danger.

A few connected this explicitly to the idea of the Other. Specifically, they highlighted the subject-positioning that was being constructed between the US and West Africa, noting the denigration of the latter to bolster the former. Some even used this to subvert the narrative. Rachel Maddow (in TRMS 2014b), as part of her argument that Ebola could easily be treated within the US, used Nigeria's success as the example to follow:

> Nigeria got Ebola from an American guy. They got it basically the same way that Dallas, Texas got Ebola. . . . And in Nigeria, they won. They were successful. They had a small outbreak in Nigeria, but they contained it. . . . Is Texas capable of doing the same thing?

In this vein, the US occupied the inferior position, yet presented itself as the superior. In drawing attention to the construction of a racialized Other, these actors were ultimately seeking to undermine the claims built on it. They sought to portray the fear surrounding the disease not as an objective appreciation of the outbreak's dangers but as one premised in prejudiced understandings of its source. It also suggested that proponents of these fear-driven discourses were purposefully playing to racist narratives, giving a more insidious spin to the claim that they were operating in self-interest (Reliable Sources 2014a; Wemple 2014a; Wickham 2014a).

And finally, the Fearbola discourse called out the prominence of intertextuality, using it to reveal how the temporal borders between possibility and plausibility had been blurred. The securitization of Ebola, as many pointed out, was not solely due to its qualities as a disease or the likelihood of infection, but its "brand" (Farhi 2014):

Public perceptions about Ebola have likely been primed by decades of movies, TV shows, and books imaging a global contagion and resulting zombie apocalypse. More than a few news stories and TV segments lately have referred to Ebola's "hot zone," which was the name of a mega-selling 1994 book about the origins of the virus.

Ebola was already "primed" for securitization because it was *known* through popular culture. Despite being far beyond the personal experience of most Americans, Ebola was not a complete unknown, but was "an ingredient in an outbreak story we're already primed to tell," regardless of how accurate that story was (Ohlheiser 2014). Fearbola proponents revealed these intertextual linkages and their power in fueling this perception of possibility and thus sought to destabilize them by differentiating them against expertise:

Zakaria: When most people think of Ebola they think, of course, about organs getting liquefied. You've seen it. You've been there? Does that ever happen?

Gupta: That's a sort of Hollywood dramatization, I believe. You know, I think it was popularized in the book *The Hot Zone*, which I think taught a lot of people about Ebola, but probably with a lot of drama as well. (Fareed Zakaria GPS 2014)

Similar to the representation of these discourses as premised on prejudiced foundations, this emphasis on intertextuality was aimed to represent the securitizing claims (particularly the AUT approach) as based on falsehood. It was particularly prominent among PGC uses of Fearbola, as it destabilized the representation of America as on the cusp of an outbreak but did not undermine the actual threat of Ebola to the US.

At its core, the Fearbola discourse did not seek to directly desecuritize the outbreak—though it was employed by some who desired to—but often functioned as a critical commentary of the securitizing discourses, occasionally in service to another. It was frequently articulated by proponents of the HWA and PGC discourses to attack the AUT approach. Obama (2014i), for instance, used the representation of the audience as capable of greater rational thought to address the calls for a travel ban. Despite the diversity in motivation, however, the four key representations within it speak to a common understanding of the outbreak and its securitized response. It was one that tapped into the audience's atavistic fears, allowing them to be misled and manipulated by self-interested and/or irresponsible elites. It drew on contextual discourses of the Dark Continent, manifesting in a reiteration of African inferiority that only served to entrench the continent's (and its people's) neglect. And it was rarely premised on an objective appreciation of the disease and the outbreak in West Africa but instead on racialized stereotypes and fictional portrayals. Ultimately, proponents of Fearbola sought to provide a counterdiscourse to all of this, whether through mockery, denigration, or simple illumination.

Conclusion

At the commencement of this book, I noted that the securitization of Ebola took multiple, competing forms. The goal of this chapter was to map the broad contours of these forms, otherwise known as the basic securitizing discourses. It was to outline and detail the general "regimes of truth" that existed throughout the political and media debate: the threats, the referent objects, the practices, the meanings of security, and the logics that underpinned them. Here, I have identified three explicitly securitizing discourses: an articulation of Ebola as a Potential Global Catastrophe that ultimately recontextualized the traditional national security approach to disease; a human-security-focused understanding of Helpless West Africa in need of American salvation; and a construction of America Under Threat from a possible Ebola pandemic. I have also noted a counterdiscourse to these securitizing claims: the Fearbola discourse, which challenged both the specific constructions at play but also—and perhaps implicitly—the underpinning logic of exceptionalism itself. Within these broad regimes of truth, nuance existed and change did occur, but they revolved around these basic nodal points.

It is important to reiterate that the goal of this chapter was not to comprehensively capture each and every articulation of the Ebola threat, even those that did fit within these basic securitizing discourses. It painted with a broader brush, identifying the key securitizing representations revealed by the analysis and the linkages between them that produced meaning. This means that nuance is missing. The changes in actor position are not evident here. While this chapter identified the actors who more commonly articulated one discursive position over others (and identified the official discourse of the Obama administration), actors did not always adhere solely to one position and their positions changed. This is particularly true for media reporters and commentators, who frequently bounced between discourses and reiterated particular representations more at particular times. Relatedly, the shift in the conditions of possibility—which representations were acceptable, expected, unaccepted, or delegitimized—is not explored here. While this chapter has outlined some of the points of intersection (and clash), it has not yet considered the play of practice between these discourses. That is the task of the next chapter.

Indeed, in outlining these basic securitizing discourses, this chapter has essentially sketched the broad boundaries of the process of securitization that occurred between them. It has identified not only the key positions but also the spaces of overlap and difference between them, where debate occurred. Some key representations were shared between discourses. There are also sites of contestation already apparent, where a basic concept (the audience, authority, exception, knowledge) is constructed in distinctly different ways. Both of these spaces are crucial. Some representations may have been shared, but the linkage to other, differing representations meant that they took on competing meanings. The subject-position of the inferior, fragile West African Other, for instance, appeared in all securitizing discourses, but took different forms in conjunction with the different representations of threat, referent object, exception, audience, knowledge, and so on. In the official PGC discourse, it resulted in a construction of West Africa as incapable of containing the outbreak and ensuring global security, necessitating US action. In the AUT discourse, it manifested in a construction of West Africans as threats themselves. And in the HWA discourse, West African Fragility connected with the position of West Africans as the referent object to represent West Africans as incapable of saving themselves but worthy of US aid. It is at these conjunctures that actors transgressed, shifted, and stood firm in their articulations of these positions. It is here that some discourses stabilized and became dominant, while others were revealed as contingent or "political." It is here, ultimately, that the securitization of Ebola truly occurred, forming a process in which the American response to the crisis formed, shifted, and ended. The next chapter now moves to explore this process in detail.

4 Securitizing Ebola

Introduction

While the previous chapter outlined how Ebola was broadly—and variously—understood as a security issue, it did not entirely explain how Ebola was *securitized*. The discourses outlined in the previous chapter were not articulated in a vacuum; they were responses to others and shifted in their key representations as they were responded to. In other words, the securitization of Ebola occurred *between* these securitizing discourses, where the interaction, contestation, and change in them shifted the boundaries of how Ebola was understood and what responses were possible. There were "successful" or dominant securitizing discourses in this process, informing the response more than others. Yet this success must be understood as relational; it was not a case of a discourse simply "winning." It was only through the destabilization, diminishment, and delegitimization of competing discourses that a particular understanding of the Ebola outbreak could come to prominence, and even this dominance was qualified and remained always unstable.

This chapter therefore finally answers the question of how exactly Ebola was securitized by exploring how the US securitization of Ebola evolved over time through this process of interaction, contestation, and discursive "play." It demonstrates that this securitization ultimately became guided by fears of a hypothetical American outbreak, where the certainty of experts was undone by a series of "what ifs" and a president's authority questioned on whether he was committed to "us" or "them." Yet these hypotheticals did not go unchallenged; early attempts to present returning health workers as threats were dismissed as immoral, efforts to enact a travel ban failed, and, even when this understanding was most prominent, its adherents were widely mocked for the irrationality and fearmongering nature of their position. What resulted was a response clearly guided by the America Under Threat (AUT) discourse but not completely driven by it, with competing approaches crucial for particular aspects of the response at particular times.

I trace this evolution through a focus on key events. Key events are "those situations where 'important facts' manifest themselves on the political and/ or the media agenda and influence the official policy-identity constellation or force the official discourse to engage with political opposition and media criticism" (Hansen 2006, 28). In essence, they are the moments that problematize the *materiality* of a discourse, necessitating their construction, reiteration, or contestation. These moments rupture what is known about an issue and become the new center of debate as discourses compete over how to interpret them. Within this case, for instance, the key events were those where either the outbreak's proximity to the US changed (returning health workers, domestic cases, internal spread) or the response changed (Obama's claiming of security and deployment of the military) or was re-contextualized (the midterm elections). The threat of Ebola, the referent object, the nature of the exception, and the best way to respond thus needed to be reasserted or reconstructed and, crucially, competing claims in these areas needed to be challenged. By examining these events as they occurred chronologically (see the introduction's overview of the outbreak and US response), we arrive at a comprehensive analysis of just how Ebola was securitized within the US, observing stability and change in how Ebola was understood as dangerous and what kind of response was deemed most appropriate.

In providing this detailed examination of the US securitization of Ebola as a process of contestation and change, this chapter ultimately reveals four specific spaces that were particularly core to Ebola's securitization and the contestation it saw: the construction of identity through the Self/Other, the production of an accepting audience, the question of authority, and the meaning and logic of security itself. These sites saw the entwining of multiple securitizing representations, such as the referent object, the threat, the audience, the securitizing actor, and emergency measures. They were also the sites of most ardent contestation. All the securitizing discourses (re)constructed a Self/Other relationship in their constructions of American and West African identities. Yet they did so in competing ways, clashing on whether the inferior West African Other was a threat to the American Self or a referent object worthy of protecting. All discourses also involved representations of "the American people" as their audience, but they competed over exactly who the American people were, what they valued, and what they wanted from their political authorities. Relatedly, three differing forms of authority (political, expert, and moral) were constructed, with debate centering on who could or should be heard and listened to, and who should not. And finally, what security itself meant and did was a key site of contestation. As the previous chapter attested, the imminence, extremity, and (un)certainty of Ebola's threat and the exceptionalism of the response were crucial to all the securitizing discourses. They were equally central to how the discourses intersected, clashed, and changed.

The Securitization of Ebola

Early Representations (March–July 2014)
Before getting to the key events, however, it is worth outlining the early representations of the outbreak for context. The outbreak entered the American consciousness around March 2014, when it was first identified and announced by the WHO. This was largely media-dominated: reporters from CNN and the *New York Times* went to Guinea to cover the story (EB:O 2014b; Gupta 2014; Newsroom 2014a; Nossiter 2014a, 2014b), and others provided periodic updates (Nightly News 2014a). From this reporting, two early representations of the outbreak—why "we" should know about it and how—became apparent.

First was the representation of Ebola as an especially "gruesome" and "scary" disease (McCoy 2014a). Its symptoms—"fever and crushing weakness [which] worsen to include diarrhea, vomiting, and internal and external bleeding" (McCoy 2014a; Nossiter 2014b; Gupta 2014)—were highlighted repeatedly, with some even asking their readers to imagine themselves suffering the effects (Gatherer 2014; see also McCoy 2014b). Infection was also emphasized, particularly its ease (Nossiter 2014b) and the fact that it spread "through the blood, secretions, and other bodily fluids" of victims (McCoy 2014a; Vladimir Duthiers, in EB:O 2014b; Lazuta 2014). In addition, many of the early representations of the outbreak stressed that the disease "had no cure" and a "90 percent" mortality rate (Erin Burnett, in EB:O 2014b; Lazuta 2014). Ebola was thus immediately represented as what Enemark

(2007, 2017b) labels a "dreaded disease," an illness that is not simply dangerous but viscerally disturbing.

The second representation presented Ebola as an African disease. In a general sense, reporters noted the previous outbreaks (predominately in the Democratic Republic of the Congo) and suggested that Ebola was simply a recurring issue that African states faced (Flanagin 2014a; McCoy 2014c; McNeil 2014a). This was more than simply a geographical linkage. The existence and spread of Ebola were understood as a distinctly "African" or "third world" phenomenon, one associated with poverty and "slums" that offer "an opportune breeding ground" for disease (Lazuta 2014), "dark jungles" rife with diseased animals (Sanjay Gupta, in EB:O 2014b), "cultural practices" replete with "misinformation and superstition" and a preference for "witch doctors" (Hogan 2014; Nossiter 2014b; Smith-Spark 2014). West Africa was immediately (re)constructed through the Dark Continent contextual discourse, with each state and its peoples represented as failing, diseased, and a source of problems for the rest of the world. This is ultimately the source of the Othering West African Fragility representation, one noted in the previous chapter as underpinning all of the securitizing discourses.

In contrast to this later use, however, these early articulations typically offered the representation as a move *against* securitization. David Quammen (2014), for instance, wrote that while people "tend to dread [Ebola] inordinately," it was not "the Next Big One, an incipient pandemic destined to circle the world," but rather "a very grim and local misery." This early media coverage presented Ebola not as a serious threat to those in West Africa, regional or global stability, or the US, but as a distant, everyday tragedy, one worth knowing and mourning, but not fearing.

The Return of Kent Brantly and Nancy Writebol (August 2014)

The diagnosis (July 23) and return (August 2 and August 6) of Kent Brantly and Nancy Writebol disrupted this representation, commencing the first key event in the US debate. Brantly and Writebol's diagnoses changed the focus and tone of the reporting, but the announcement of their return was a defining moment. It was quickly summarized by reporters as "Ebola . . . coming to the US" (Wilson, J. 2014). CNN broadcasted Brantly's arrival and transport to Emory live with a running commentary (Newsroom 2014b), while the helicopter images of him walking slowly into the hospital in full personal protective equipment were repeatedly shown by both print and television media.

This coverage never used the term *security*, but it did introduce an equally distinctive term, one that invoked the exceptionalism of security while stretching it temporally and spatially. Brantly's arrival (and the impending one of Writebol) was repeatedly referred to as a possible *risk* to the US:

> It's a big step. You take the risk of moving somebody with the virus that kills 90 percent of the people who get it. A virus with no cure and no vaccine into the United States, exposing possibly others to it.[1] (Erin Burnett, in EB:O 2014c)

Brantly and Writebol were not depicted as inevitable harbingers of a pandemic. Rather, they were represented as glimpses at its possibility. Media figures pondered whether the residents around the hospital or the medical personnel within it were at risk or presented one themselves (Nightly News 2014b; MTP 2014a; SRBB 2014a). Assertions that Emory was prepared were qualified with the fact that "the risk is not zero" and "mistakes do happen, don't they?" (Chris Wallace, in FNS 2014a). This ostensible risk, moreover, was represented not as the fear of these commentators, but as that of the audience: "you know, some people are—are concerned and perhaps rightly so, perhaps not, that there is Ebola now coming to the United States" (Willie Geist, in Today 2014a). This was the first appearance of the AUT discourse.

While this AUT understanding of Brantly and Writebol quickly became the dominant interpretation, it was just as quickly challenged. Notably, this discussion continued to gravitate around the idea of risk (or security), focusing on just *how* it was constructed and whether this was apt. One important challenge centered on the form of knowledge underpinning these claims: possibility over probability. Some starkly dismissed this as conjecture on the basis of ignorance:

> There is a very simple test for how worried you should be, you at home, should be, about contracting the Ebola virus. . . . So here's the test. Are you exchanging bodily fluids with someone who has contracted Ebola? No? Settle down. (Ezra Klein, in All In 2014a)

Other media commentators and key government officials offered more gentle rebukes. In a hearing before the Subcommittee on Africa, Global Health, Global Human Rights, and International Organizations on the outbreak, Frieden (in CFA 2014a, 11) asserted, "it is important to keep in mind" that while "we don't have medications that can cure [Ebola]," "we do know how to control it, and we can stop it." Certainty was thus stressed as a response to the speculation occurring: Ebola may be a "scary disease," but it was one that was *known* (Frieden, in MTP 2014a).

Critics also reframed this linkage of Brantly and Writebol to risk, presenting it as a selfish prioritization of own's own perceived risk over Brantly and Writebol's actual risk of death. Extreme examples of this were highlighted, such as a tweet by future president Donald Trump (2014)—"The U.S. cannot allow EBOLA infected people back. People that go to far away places to help out are great—but must suffer the consequences!"—and Ann Coulter's (2014) rant about Brantly's "idiotic" efforts in "disease-ridden cesspools."[2] Critics employed this and other quotes to reconstruct the wider AUT claim surrounding Brantly and Writebol as equivalent:

> News and social media portrayed them as some kind of pathogenic juggernauts who might carry a horrible condition to our shores. This unthinking reaction is the opposite of what is called for. These workers should be given a heartfelt salute for having the courage to serve on the front lines of a battle as fierce as any in the world today. (WP 2014a)

Brantly and Writebol were represented here as archetypes of the Heroic Health Worker: "inspiring role models," putting "their lives on the line to stop a viral freight train that is picking up speed" (Siegel 2014).[3] They were thus ascribed a kind of moral authority, one that reframed them and their actions as noble and unimpeachable. Accordingly, to suggest that they were to blame for their own infection, or for bringing Ebola to the US was "blaming the Ebola victim" (Rosenthal 2014).

In addition to disputing their representation as dangerous, the moral authority ascribed to Brantly and Writebol also reframed their cause—aiding West Africa—as just. They thus provided "a good wakeup call for us" regarding the long-neglected outbreak in West Africa (Sheri Fink, in Newsroom 2014c). This was a form of the Helpless West Africa (HWA) discourse that was constructed *against* the AUT approach. Rather than simply focusing on the West African referent object, it had to engage the prevailing representation of the US as holding this subject-position. It did so through juxtaposing representations of the two. The US, it was repeatedly noted, was not West Africa. It was "high-tech" (Charles Krauthammer, in SRBB 2014b), with "modern" (Nancy Snyderman, in MTP 2014a) facilities that West African states—"among the poorest and most war-racked" (NYT 2014c)—simply lacked (Ken Isaacs, in CFA 2014a, 52). The US was "advanced" (Sanjay Gupta, in EB:O 2014c), while (West) Africa was constituted by "primitive deathbeds" (Graham 2014). This temporal differentiation of advanced (US)/backward (Africa) was thus linked to representations of capability/incapability and, ultimately, safe/unsafe. The US, constructed as the advanced, capable Self, was thus not truly at risk: "The idea that they can't be brought back to the country by people who are clearly very qualified and know how to handle the situation . . . the real tragedy and epidemic that is going on is not in the United States. It's in Africa" (Powers, in SRBB 2014b).

This HWA reframing of the referent object had mixed levels of success. On the one hand, it was successful in altering the ethical boundaries of the discussion. West Africans not only returned to focus but were understood as Others worthy of protection. CNN sent reporters back to West Africa. Questions arose around the differences in treatment and emphasis. Erin Burnett (in EB:O 2014e), for instance, asked why experimental treatments provided to Brantly and Writebol were not more available:

> I know it is miraculous, untested, risky, but what about everyone else? Nearly a thousand have died. All of them Africans. Suddenly two white Americans get the disease and suddenly all of the stops get pulled out.

A short debate sparked around the ethics of treatment disparity. Some saw providing untested treatments to West Africans as an ethical obligation (see Dionne 2014). Others worried it was a violation of ethics concerning informed consent (see Seay 2014). Franklin Graham (2014) of Samaritan's Purse, meanwhile, was enraged by what the debate suggested about Brantly and Writebol's worthiness to receive the treatment. Eventually, the WHO (2014) convened a meeting of bioethicists to decide on using experimental treatments in West Africa.

Yet even this success was limited. The AUT discourse shifted, but not too far. The representation of Brantly and Writebol as risks increasingly seemed untenable, yet the concern with potential contagion remained. Media commentary started to reframe the two as the "best-case scenario" of Ebola in the US: immediate isolation, continuous surveillance, and specialist treatment. This was then juxtaposed with a new threat:

> Bringing Ebola to the United States on purpose for the plan to quarantine and treat the patient, that's one thing. But having someone just arrived in the US with the virus, that's totally different. And it's public health experts' worst fear. (Brooke Baldwin, in Newsroom 2014d)

The threat became the hypothetical traveler: the body moving Ebola from the "hot zone" to the US, with travelers "unknowingly carrying this disease . . . [into] an emergency room at a hospital in this country" (Betsy McCaughey and Neil Cavuto, in YWNC 2014a).

More specifically, they speculated about the prospect of an *African* traveler. Reporting returned to the coverage of Ebola as an "African problem," running rampant through the "worst slums in the world" (McCoy 2014f; see also Larimer 2014a), where residents engage in "looting sprees" (Paye-Layleh 2014) and "use the beaches as public bathrooms" (McCoy 2014f). Consequently, the Hypothetical Traveler progressively became the "hypothetical African traveler." In some cases, (West) African bodies were not the only fear. In a widely circulated article in *Newsweek*, two reporters suggested that West African immigrant communities were smuggling "bushmeat contaminated with the virus . . . into the US in luggage," threatening an outbreak (Flynn and Scutti 2014). Attempts to keep the West African referent central thus sat alongside representations that presented them as the dangerous Other, whether they physically resided within the affected states or not. Ultimately, underpinning these claims was the Dark Continent and its central narrative: (West) African inferiority as directly dangerous to the US.

The AUT discourse also evolved in response to the challenges to its speculative basis of knowledge. Uncertainty had been key in early articulations of the AUT discourse, yet it remained unstated what exactly was uncertain. Critics' responses thus emphasized what was known, and while this diminished particular claims, it also encouraged a more explicit articulation of where the gaps (supposedly) were: in how Ebola was transmitted. Rep. Chris Smith (in Newsroom 2014e), for instance, told CNN:

> I and others . . . are very concerned about others who might come here by way of a flight, who have a slight fever and the next thing you know, they have Ebola. Then, everyone they have been in contact with, where there was touch or some kind of exchange of bodily fluid . . . we don't know, frankly, and I think it's pretty clear that it's not passed on by way of air or breathing or getting close in that way. [But] the jury is always out on other ways of transmission.

Accordingly, AUT proponents were not "overreacting" but being cautious: "it's always best to err on the side of worrying a little bit" when "no-one seem[s] to know" (Daniel Bongino, in YWNC 2014a). Speculating on the possibilities, even when these possibilities had been disproved by the CDC, was necessary. In fact, some even suggested that it may have even been necessary *because* the CDC said it was unlikely, pointing to past mistakes and asking, "how are we supposed to trust you now, after there were such big safety lapses back then?" (Bret Baier, in SRBB 2014c; see also Today 2014a). CDC expertise and authority were represented as tenuous, their knowledge flawed, and thus a threat in itself. In this way, the AUT discourse evolved to not only contest the Potential Global Catastrophe (PGC) and HWA representation of certainty but also to contest the very basis of expert authority on which certainty might built.

These points of contestation and alignment came to a head in the question of the exception. Proponents of the AUT and HWA discourses shared the position that the outbreak was a matter of urgent, exceptional danger, urging further action. They also shared the perspective that key security actors—the CDC, the WHO, and the Obama administration, particularly—did not completely recognize the gravity of the situation. For AUT proponents, particularly politicians, true sovereign action was absent: "I [am] concerned that no-one [at the White House] could tell me who was in charge within the administration on this issue" (Frank Wolf, in CFA 2014a, 7). HWA proponents were equally concerned with how the outbreak had "laid bare how unprepared the United States and other advanced countries are to protect and treat thousands of Africans whose lives are threatened by an extremely dangerous virus" (NYT 2014b). Political authority was thus also contested.

This representation was somewhat apt. The Obama administration seemed to largely dismiss the exception. As Obama (2014a) himself outlined it during a press conference, the prime issue was not an exceedance of "normality," but the lack of an appropriate one: "the countries that have been affected are the first to admit that what's happened here is, is that their public health systems have been overwhelmed." The appropriate response was thus one of "surging resources" already available within the CDC and USAID to "help these countries accomplish" the basics of (normal) public health. Yet in making this claim, the Obama administration missed that the outbreak was already being constructed as an exceptional danger. A disparity opened between this position and the growing public understanding of the outbreak. This was compounded by expert authorities, namely Frieden (in AC360 2014c) after a trip to West Africa where he depicted it as "an absolute emergency" and Médecins Sans Frontières president Dr. Joanne

Liu (2014) during a rebuke to the UN that "the response has been too little, too late." As a later Department of Defense analysis described it, this formed a "tipping point" in the response, one that sparked the next key event (JCOA 2016, 5).

Within just this one key event, we can observe the centrality of the four key sites outlined in this chapter's introduction. The West African Other and the American Self were ascribed different meanings, linked to representations of threat and referent to produce two different subject-positions for West Africa (the victim in need of aid [and pharmaceutical salvation] and the hypothetical traveler) and the US (the capable responder and the vulnerable referent). The audience and its ostensible concern were widely employed by media figures to justify their questions regarding possible threat, but experts also sought to answer these questions with reference to rational thought and certainty. Authority too became important, with Brantly and Writebol defended as moral authorities, the CDC both upheld as the "experts" to answer speculation and challenged as a flawed institution, and the president's actions questioned for whether they were appropriately sovereign. And ultimately, underpinning all of this were competing understandings of security itself: risk and possibility against imminence and certainty. Accordingly, Brantly and Writebol's return set the stage for the events to come.

The Securitizing Moves of President Obama (September 2014)

September brought the intervention of the sovereign. Obama made what have since been called his "securitizing speech acts": his speeches to the CDC and UN justifying an expanded federal response. I add to Obama's "securitizing moves"—typically referring to a speech to the CDC (September 16) and two to the UN (September 24 and 25)—an appearance on NBC's *Meet the Press* (September 7). While not notable for international audiences, Obama's widely requoted[4] interview on NBC was the first time he asserted the outbreak was a "national security priority" (MTP 2014b). As outlined in the first chapter, this framing of securitizing moves and speech acts is problematic. It suggests that securitization solely occurred here and can be analyzed from just this moment. Yet, as the previous discussion on Brantly and Writebol's return demonstrates, securitizing discourses had already been articulated and reiterated, with four key sites for this construction and contestation apparent. Obama's speeches and interview did not start this process of securitization, but they did disrupt the materiality of it (as key events do). They did so through explicitly connecting it to the label of security.

Across these four moves, Obama provided a clear articulation of the PGC discourse. Ebola was a threat to "public health systems" and "economic growth," risking a "regional crisis" which could "quickly become [a] global threat" (Obama 2014e). This necessitated an extraordinary response: Operation United Assistance, the first US military operation to respond to a disease outbreak (JCOA 2016, v). Obama (2014b) depicted this as the US "tak[ing] leadership on this to provide the kinds of capabilities that only America has, and to mobilize the world in ways that only America can do." Stopping such a threat to global security was the "burden" that the world's superpower had to bear, and (true) Americans "welcome these responsibilities; we don't shy away from them" (Obama 2014c).

Yet while these speeches all served to articulate and rearticulate the core PGC discourse, two noteworthy differences existed between some of them, which speak to both the nuances of the PGC discourse and the evolution of it in the public sphere. The first concerned the possibility of mutation. In his *Meet the Press* appearance, Obama (in MTP 2014b) outlined one of the threats as "the prospect that the virus mutates." This concern is missing, however, from his later speeches to the CDC and UN. The reason may lie in what occurred in between. On September 12, an opinion piece by prominent infectious disease expert Michael Osterholm (2014b) was published in the *New York Times* which suggested that virologists were hiding their fears that Ebola "could mutate to become transmissible through the air." Osterholm's established position as an infectious disease expert saw the suggestion widely reiterated and defended (Cohen 2014), including within a congressional hearing (Betty McCollum, in CFA 2014b, 14). Public health figures, including Anthony Fauci, disputed the likelihood of such a "terrifying scenario" and criticized Osterholm for fostering "a public distrust in scientists" with his claim that experts were keeping quiet about this threat (Larimer 2014b; TSR 2014b). The absence of mutation from Obama's next, more substantive, securitizing moves can thus perhaps be observed as an attempt to sidestep this contested issue. Notably, this returns us to the debates around risk, knowledge, and experts that appeared during Brantly and Writebol's return: the suggestion of mutation was one of speculation from uncertainty while critics countered by relying on what was known and understood about the virus, and both positions relied on—and challenged—expert authority.

The second difference concerns what replaced this anxiety regarding mutation in the later speeches: an alignment with the HWA discourse and an emphasis on the West African referent. Ebola was "wiping out whole families," turning "simply acts of love and comfort . . . into potentially fatal acts" and it was this that necessitated "an urgent, strong and coordinated international response" (Obama 2014e). This was the exception as produced by the HWA discourse. Yet Obama (2014e) then dismissed this as the "health crisis," with the security element as "more than" this. In essence, he borrowed the HWA exception to amplify the outbreak's exceptional nature, but he does not locate security's meaning here. This label was confined solely to the potential catastrophe: the economic shocks, political collapse, and military destabilization of the region.

Obama's label of national security was described as a "game-changer" (Laurie Garrett, in Sun and Eilperin 2014). Yet, in a demonstration of the signifying capacity of security, what precisely it changed was open to interpretation. Some simply reproduced Obama's securitizing representations as an objective description (Nancy Snyderman, in Nightly News 2014c). Others expanded and contextualized it through interviewing health workers, other government officials, the CDC, Médecins Sans Frontières, and the WHO (AC360 2014d; Nakamura 2014a; Newsroom 2014g; TSR 2014b, 2014d), providing it a veneer of expert authority. Others, however, reframed Obama's claim to security. Some suggested that Obama's key message was one more in line with the HWA discourse. Here, certain quotes were reiterated—"these men and women and children are just sitting, waiting to die, right now" and "the world still has an opportunity to save countless lives"—while others denoting the more traditional security approach were left out, effectively reproducing Obama's speeches as "an impassioned call" to save West Africa (Deloffre 2014; Sun and Eilperin 2014). Ultimately, such claims (and the lack of dispute from officials) were a continuation of the HWA and PGC alignment, which spoke to Obama's success in drawing on the HWA exception. Yet this alignment required differences to be smoothed over, which was possible when the debate remained relatively abstract, but quickly became problematic when security's meaning and practice were actually considered.

Indeed, practice was the central site of contestation. On the one hand, Obama broadly fulfilled the expected role of commander in chief of the Indispensable Nation, with the proposed deployment of troops not only appropriate, but an example of benevolent American power saving the world. Even those who critiqued it shared this understanding of exception and the need for emergency measures (WP 2014c; John Boehner, quoted in Sun and Eilperin 2014). On the other hand, the differing understandings of security demanded differing responses. An immediate threat to West Africa denoted a different solution to that plausibly posed to global stability. Specifically, were the "boots on the ground" the boots that were truly needed? Some lamented that the US was not supplying the "actual doctor and nurse boots on the ground" that were needed for an adequate response, perhaps out of a concern with the risk to American lives over the actual threat to West African ones (Elizabeth Cohen, in Newsroom 2014f). Obama, in other words, did not see the danger as exceptional enough.

The AUT discourse also aligned and contested with this newly formalized PGC response. Yet it did so in two forms. The first was largely a reiteration of that proposed during Brantly and Writebol's return to the US: the threat as infected outsiders, particularly the "200,000 Africans from countries hosting the deadly Ebola virus who hold temporary visas to the United States," and the need for containment (Andrea Tantaros, in The Five 2014a). Obama's early appearance (and Osterholm) added a new flavoring to this specific threat:

> The other thing, which is unstated because you don't want to start a panic, is that it is possible—extremely unlikely but possible—that the virus mutates and becomes more easy to transmit, perhaps even by respiratory means. . . . So it's because of that remote possibility . . . that we want to make sure that it stays in West Africa, and deploying the military and all of our resources is a good thing to do. (Charles Krauthammer, in SRBB 2014e)

The significance of the mutation linkage cannot be understated. The topic came up no fewer than four times during the second hearing of the Subcommittee on Africa, Global Health, Global Human Rights, and International Organizations held on September 17, from both Republican and Democrat members (CFA 2014b, 65, 67, 71, 72). It was mentioned alongside Obama's later speeches—despite the topic being absent from them—as the "nightmare scenario" they were aimed to prevent (Korte and Szabo 2014). This effectively merged the AUT concern regarding the risk to the American populace with the PGC threat to global spread. The potential for mutation—and in ways that concern us, such as airborne transmission—meant that it was important to act in West Africa now to contain the disease both geographically and biologically. In this vein, for such commentators, the practical response suited their construction of security.

Again, however, this did not mean an easy alliance. Some insisted that while emergency action was appreciated, more important—and necessary—security practices were not being implemented. One area of direct concern was the insistence on safety testing in pharmaceutical development:

> I guess I am just a little disappointed, Dr. Borio, to hear about a clinical hold. . . . Instead of talking about clinical holds, let us talk about clinical trials. . . . There is a broad understanding at the Food and Drug Administration that this is no ordinary time, correct? (Michael Burgess, in CFA 2014b, 74)

This was the exception as proposed by the AUT discourse: the (possible, future) threat was so overwhelming as to warrant the closure of normal regulatory process. It also demanded a central sovereign figure, with senators demanding to know "who's in charge of all of that" (John Boozman, in CHELP 2014, 42). Again, these debated constructions of security's meaning and logic entwined with those of authority. Obama's political authority was drawn into focus, with critics representing him as ceding the space to bureaucrats, medical figures, and, perhaps even worse, the WHO (Gerson 2014a; Strain 2014).

The second manifestation of the AUT discourse was that of dismissal. This form of the AUT discourse insisted that Ebola may be a concern, but it was not the *security* concern Obama was making it out to be. Indeed, it was even a misplacement of the exception, a particularly egregious issue when more obvious issues of security were ignored:

> Here's what I'd like him to do. I'd like him to step up and say "we're doing everything we can to eradicate ISIS." Yes, Ebola is going to be a problem. It's going to be—it could be a pandemic, and we're going to do everything we can. But let's focus on the most pressing thing to the United States. In my opinion, the most dangerous thing to the United States right now is terrorism. (Eric Bolling, in The Five 2014a)

Evident here is also a concern with the exceptionalism embodied in the deployment of the military. There is almost an equivalence between them being drawn: to deploy the military is to decide an exception, and to decide an exception demands deploying the military. Having one without the other is thus to politicize both.

Obama's introduction of the security signifier did not drastically alter this debate, but it did force an evolution of it. The three key securitizing discourses persisted but changed in accordance with this new "reality," aligning and challenging one another. Again, the four sites of identity, audience, authority, and security were key, but some were more important here than others. Particularly central to these claims and the disputes between them was a recognition that the exceptionalism of security provided several political possibilities—some more extreme than others—that the government had chosen not to embrace. This choice, and the contestation around it, was based in how the outbreak's threat was understood (and whose knowledge we should listen to), whose lives were worth defending, and to what lengths "we" were prepared to go to defend them. If the outbreak had continued in its current form, the tenuous alignments and undercurrent of contestation might have sufficed. Yet the very last day of September 2014 offered the material challenge to beat all material challenges: a Liberian national named Thomas Eric Duncan tested positive for Ebola in Dallas, Texas.

Thomas Eric Duncan, Nina Pham, and Amber Joy Vinson (Early October 2014)

Following the announcement of Duncan's diagnosis, Frieden (in CDC 2014a) gave a press conference in which he sought to give meaning to the event. He did so by linking Duncan, his illness, and his treatment to the PGC narrative. The case reflected "the ongoing spread of Ebola in Liberia and West Africa" and the fact that "we are all connected." Frieden was not simply reiterating the PGC discourse. He was sharpening its boundaries against the AUT discourse. Duncan was both the prime example of the threat in West Africa, the need to act there and stop the outbreak, but he was also the "test case" to demonstrate that the US would "stop it here" (CDC 2014a). Frieden (in CDC 2014a) repeatedly emphasized what was known, certain, and controllable about this case, asserting that "Ebola only spreads through direct contact" and that the US health system had "tried and true protocol[s]." Claims against this, therefore, were a denial of what was known, and therefore irrational, unscientific, and fear-driven.

None of this, of course, stopped AUT proponents from challenging this narrative. Indeed, directly following Frieden's opening statement, CNN's live coverage cut back to the studio for Wolf Blitzer (in TSR 2014c) to express his alarm that "there could have been other people who were infected, if you will, over these days since this individual showed symptoms." October 1 saw television coverage opening with:

> It's here: the major fear tied to the first person diagnosed with Ebola in the U.S. Will it spread? That patient now in isolation in Dallas while officials attempt to track down anyone who came in contact with him. So how concerned should we be? (Matt Lauer, in Today 2014c)

This was a direct contestation of Frieden's emphasis on probability and certainty. It was an argument that the possible and unknown needed to be prioritized. Fox News's Bill O'Reilly (in TOF 2014a) affirmed that he "believe[d]" the CDC director when he insisted that Duncan was not contagious during his flights. But, as he followed, "why take the chance"? Was it "unreasonable" to worry about the possibility of being infected on a flight (Tamron Hall, in Today 2014c)? Was it "wrong to be a little worried, maybe even a little panicked about whether our health care system is equipped to handle something that's been so destructive halfway across the world" (Steve Kornacki, in TRMS 2014a)? For these commentators, the consequence of an Ebola outbreak in the US was so great that the fear of it outweighed its minuscule likelihood.

Again, this was a construction of security as risk merged with the Schmittian exception. It saw the threat as extreme but temporally stretched with an uncertain knowledge base. This all occurred through the construction of security through *speculation*. Media reporting became imaginative, focused on the unknowns. Reporters highlighted the times in which Duncan's precise whereabouts were uncertain, drawing into focus the figures who might have occupied these spaces (schoolchildren, members of the community) and how their possible infection might have occurred (Early Start 2014c; Berman and Nutt 2014; Newsroom 2014h; TSR 2014d). They questioned Frieden's statements. What did we really know? How much should we trust these claims?

> When talking about this Ebola case in the US, you said, quote "There is no doubt in my mind that we will stop it here." And I think anybody hearing those words hopes you're right. But how can you be so sure? How can you be sure that you've identified everyone that this patient came into contact with after he became symptomatic? (Matt Lauer, in Today 2014c)

Once again, reporters framed these questions and imaginative scenarios as simply the worries of the audience. Duncan became the empirical test case that proved the danger of certainty. He had "lied" to get into the country, demonstrating the problems with the "honor system" of screenings (Steve Scalise, in YWNC 2014c; see also Onishi and Mouawad 2014). The missteps of the hospital he was treated at—namely the misdiagnosis of Duncan when he first appeared in the ER—were offered as "proof that things are not foolproof" (Tamron Hall, in Today 2014c) and that the US had "flunked the readiness test" (Betsy McCaughey, in YWNC 2014b). The danger was thus no longer just the hypothetical (spread from Duncan), but the failure to adequately respond to it. All was uncertain, and therefore all was threatening.

This was not only a reproduction of the threat but also (and perhaps more crucially) a reproduction of the PGC and HWA discourses. Their claim that the threat was known and could be contained was, at best, "overly optimistic and full of misleading assurances" (Dausey 2014), and, at worst, outright dangerous:

> Now, do I know it's going to happen? No, nobody knows. But it is absolutely a mistake to take a [position of] political correctness and say they know with certainty it's not going to spread and, as a consequence, so play down fears that we don't take precaution. (Rand Paul, quoted in Killough 2014)

Indeed, to claim certainty was "political correctness." Obama and the CDC were "so concerned with avoiding panic that they're willing to say anything, even if it shreds their credibility" (Dausey 2014). Obama was even suggested to be "thinking globally instead of patriotically," absconding on his "first duty" to "protect and secure the people 100 percent" (Sean Hannity and Pat Buchanan, in Hannity 2014b). Their response was not objective, but a political interpretation, a prioritization of normal politics over the (apolitical) exception Ebola posed. The construction of risk was thus infused with one of authority, challenging the political authority of Obama and the expert authority of the CDC.

Despite suggestions that they would hold firm against the rising dominance of the AUT discourse, some accommodation was apparent in PGC responses. Obama's (2014g) prepared remarks increasingly differentiated the "national security priority" of Ebola in the US from "just a humanitarian issue or a public health issue." Shifting rhetoric was matched by practice. October 8 saw "enhanced screening" implemented at five international airports, those which oversaw approximately 97 percent of travel from West Africa. It was presented by the secretary of homeland security, Jeh Johnson (in CDC 201b), as evidence that they "will continue to assess the risk of the spread of Ebola into the United States, and take additional measures, as necessary, to protect the American people." Such screening, however, would not have detected Thomas Eric Duncan, who did not show symptoms until after his arrival and passed the questioning of screeners. Some thus labeled these measures as mere security theater (Drezner 2014c). The CDC later confirmed this in their own evaluations of their response, describing these "enhancements" as "in response" to "demands . . . from some political leaders and members of the public" (Cohen et al. 2016, 58, 60).

Indeed, this was not a drastic alteration of the PGC discourse but a rearticulation of it that permitted it to "answer" the AUT discourse. It was a response, in other words, to the fact that the AUT discourse had shifted the boundaries of the debate to gravitate around the possible risk to the US from West Africans. Even while proponents of this approach disagreed with this framing, they had to speak and act within its confines. Take, for example, Frieden's announcement of the enhanced screenings. He again insisted that "nothing we can do will get us to absolute zero risk until we end the Ebola epidemic in West Africa," but he still articulated his actions as "further protect[ing] the health of Americans" (CDC 2014b). Similarly, while Obama's (2014e) answers to reporters' questions indicated that he was not able to completely abandon the "children on the streets dying of this disease," his prepared remarks still reiterated that the focus was on protecting the US.

It was at this point that Nina Pham, one of Duncan's attending nurses, tested positive for Ebola. Another nurse, Amber Joy Vinson, followed closely behind. The quick succession of new diagnoses, as well as the revelation that Vinson had traveled via plane to Ohio and back, came as an avalanche of bad news that only seemed to confirm the AUT discourse's representation of the threat, authorities, and knowledge. Or, at least, this is how this event was represented. Vinson was depicted as a Typhoid Mary-type figure (Chris Matthews, in Hardball 2014c) and Frieden and Obama were again depicted as having prioritized "reassurance" over the "truth" (Chuck Todd, in MTP 2014c). Pham and Vinson were thus a confirmation that the "fears Ebola could spread . . . are not irrational" (Greta van Susteren, in Greta 2014b).

Again, accommodation was evident, but qualified. In his announcement, Frieden noted that "the existence of the first case of Ebola spread in the US changes some things," but he quickly added that it doesn't change others:

It doesn't change the fact that we know how Ebola spreads. It doesn't change the fact that it's possible to treat Ebola safely. But it does change, substantially, how we approach it. (CDC 2014c)

This approach required a "rethink," in Frieden's words. More specifically, it was announced on October 15 that the CDC would be sending specialized teams—what Obama (2014h) labeled "a SWAT team, essentially, from the CDC"—to aid with US Ebola patients. The guidelines on what constituted adequate personal protective equipment were "tightened" on October 20 (CDC 2014d). None of this constituted a substantive backtrack in the sense that the threat was altered or the emergency measures were fundamentally flawed. Yet this was how it was depicted: "last week we were getting these reassurances and we were hearing repeatedly about how hard it was to catch Ebola [and] today he is talking about having to rethink our entire approach" (Steve Hayes, in SRBB 2014f).

Frieden's authority as an expert, challenged before, was now almost entirely dismissed. During a hearing of the Subcommittee on Oversight and Investigation on October 16, Frieden was the main target of nearly every round of questions (CEC 2014a). He was presented as politically contaminated ("is this your opinion or does someone also advise you, someone within the Administration, any other agencies?"), not apologetic enough about his "mistakes" ("I appreciate Dr. Daniel Varga's statement of honesty that we made mistakes. I didn't hear that from any of you, and that troubles me."), and, just as crucially, not as certain as the American people supposedly hoped he was:

You know, I want to—one of my main concerns, Dr. Frieden, is that we don't know what we don't know. Throughout testimony and questioning today, I have heard you say multiple times "I don't know the details of this, I don't know the details of that," and I think what the American people are wanting is some assurance that somebody does know the details. (Bill Johnson, in CEC 2014a: 144–145)

In the media, Frieden's critics labeled him a "liar," a "propagandist," and a "puppet" for the Obama administration (Bill O'Reilly, in TOF 2014c). Even those sympathetic described him as having made "the worst possible action" in this political battle: "in an effort to keep the public calm, the CDC pretended to know more about Ebola than it actually does" (Berezow 2014). And, in perhaps the strongest indicator of how diminished Frieden's authority was, the White House itself criticized him and sought to distance the president from him. A story in the New York Times quoted "senior officials and aides" in describing Obama as "visibly angry" with Frieden and the CDC for misleading him (Shear and Landler 2014).

Obama too was represented as a failing political authority. More specifically, he was not acting as the sovereign, absconding from his decisional power right as it was deemed necessary. The question of who was in charge came back to the fore, framed as a need of the fearful and helpless audience, who sought "an appointed John Wayne dude . . . to get things under control" (Metzgar 2013; see also Eilperin 2014a; Rubin 2014a). Initially, the Obama administration resisted such calls, but on October 17 it announced the designation of Ron Klain as the Ebola response coordinator or, as he was immediately known: the Ebola czar. Klain, as both his critics and admirers presented him, was a seasoned political operative, a specialist at organizing, governing, managing, and centralizing. Difference, however, lay in what kind of job Klain's management acumen was being squeezed into. For PGC and HWA proponents, the role was one of intergovernmental coordination and oversight, or "crossing all the t's and dotting all the i's" (Obama, quoted in Eilperin 2014b). Klain was "smart, aggressive, and levelheaded; exactly the qualities we need in a czar" (Chuck Schumer, quoted in Eilperin and Nakamura 2014). For critics of the AUT persuasion, however, the job was one of knowing and guiding the medical response, ostensibly a Frieden replacement. Klain was therefore not only unqualified, but a "political hack" (Geraldo Rivera, in TOF 2014d; Reince Priebus, in FNS 2014b), a "mouthpiece" of the government (Bill O'Reilly, in TOF 2014d; Ted Cruz, in SOTU 2014b), and yet another piece of evidence that the Obama administration was "unserious" about the threat of Ebola to the US (Cruz 2014b).

As these shifts in both the response and the justification of it demonstrate, the AUT discourse was clearly dominant at this point in time. Yet it was not so dominant as to completely control the narrative. In fact, it was at this point that its key representations were most explicitly challenged, as the Fearbola counterdiscourse came into ascendance. The fears of an American outbreak were increasingly reproduced as irrational, an "indecent" and excessively emotional response, with "a flood of recriminations, political showboating and panicked overreactions" (Schmemann 2014b). Commentators variously highlighted "the racial component of all this, the arrogance, the first world versus the third world" (Miles O'Brien, in Reliable Sources 2014a), interviewed psychologists to explore this "instinctual panic" (Carey 2014), and offered anecdotes of racialized abuse and threats to health workers (Sack et al. 2014; Sanburn 2014). The sources of this fear, however, differed. The media (Miles O'Brien, in Reliable Sources 2014a), Republican "political opportunism" (Steinhauer 2014; Al Sharpton, in PN 2014a), and the audience itself were all blamed (Chuck Todd, in MTP 2014c; Brooks and Collins 2014). Despite the differences, these claims formed a powerful counterdiscourse, a crucial counterpoint to a debate that was otherwise lost in the battle between the (PGC) Obama administration and its (AUT) opponents.

The case of Thomas Eric Duncan should be remembered for its tragedy. Duncan's death might have been avoided had he been diagnosed correctly or his symptoms monitored more closely. Some parts of the media did give respectful attention to this, particularly in allowing his fiancé a voice (Brown and Phillip 2014). For the most part, however, Duncan was subsumed into the broader debate around Ebola's securitization. He was the hypothetical (West) African traveler made real or a marker of why the US needed to act with more urgency within West Africa. He was a justification for the audience's fears or a reminder of why they were irrational. He symbolized both the unknown and the expected, as well as the hubris of authorities and the very reason why they were necessary. He was ultimately both threat and victim, but the representation of the former was especially successful. Around Thomas Eric Duncan, the debates around the Self/Other, the audience, authority, and security resolidified, and the securitization of Ebola shifted to align closer to the securitizing discourse that saw this danger as an African one to the fearful American people.

Tracing Craig Spencer and Quarantining Kaci Hickox (Late October 2014)

It was in this context of AUT dominance that Craig Spencer was diagnosed with Ebola in New York City. Spencer had recently returned from treating Ebola patients in West Africa with Médecins Sans Frontières. When he detected a fever on October 23, he isolated himself and reported his symptoms. He was admitted to Bellevue Hospital, placed into isolation, and diagnosed that night. Spencer, in other words, did everything he was supposed to do. However, in the week prior to becoming contagious, he had traveled around New York City and spent evenings with friends, including at a bowling alley the night before he fell ill. He had not, as a "law enforcement source" told CNN, quarantined himself, which led "investigators" to take this case "very seriously" (Newsroom 2014i). Accordingly, Spencer was immediately framed as the next "hypothetical traveler," the next Thomas Eric Duncan.

Spencer's diagnosis, like Duncan's, was announced at a press conference by mayor of New York City Bill de Blasio, New York governor Andrew Cuomo, and others (including Frieden) who all sought to define the case (NYC 2014). Here, however, speakers immediately went on the defensive. The overwhelming message from the authorities was that Spencer was a success and would continue to be a success. "Success," of course, was defined by the AUT discourse as it had dominated the Duncan debate. He was identified and isolated (unlike Duncan). His contacts would be traced and isolated (unlike Duncan). And he would be treated by health workers prepared for the task (unlike Duncan). Frieden (in NYC 2014) even summarized this response as one that "absolutely minimizes risk." Again, while this was the same claim that the risk could be managed, it had shifted from being a dismissal of risk as threat to the centralizing of it to the response.

As with the other cases, the media focused again on what remained unknown and possible. Spencer's movements were traced by both newspaper and television reports, with lists of each location he had visited and how he had traveled to and from there (ABC News 2014; CBS News 2014; EB:O 2014f). Reports also focused on the precise symptoms Spencer was said to have, with a particular focus being on the fact that he noted "feel[ing] a bit sluggish" before he reported himself (Poppy Harlow, in Early Start 2014d). Competing information was also highlighted: an anonymous health worker at Bellevue Hospital was quoted as saying that Spencer "seemed very sick" and questioned "why he had not gone to the hospital earlier" (Santora 2014a). For media commentators, this opened the possibility for multiple spaces of contagion:

> But it's what happened before that, when he had this symptom of fatigue which was yesterday and the day before that, of course, many here in the media and the public might be concerned about. That's because he rode the A-train, the L-train. He went to the high line. He went jogging. He went to a restaurant. He went to a bowling alley in Williamsburg. (Sharon Crowley, in Hannity 2014c)

Of course, as interviewed medical experts and even the news anchors themselves repeatedly noted, spread at any of these points was highly unlikely. But the possibility, as they argued, needed to be considered because the audience ostensibly demanded it: "You can understand the fear. You don't want to be dismissive of the fear." (Sanjay Gupta, in TSR 2014e). The representation of the audience as perhaps irrational but understandably fearful became dominant.

While Spencer was positioned as similar to Duncan in terms of threat, crucial differences also appeared, complicating this construction. Namely, Spencer was not African. He could not be positioned as an Other, one outside of the US's moral community, even by those most communitarian in their perspective. Spencer was an American health worker returning home. Indeed, he was a "committed and responsible" man with "an affinity for helping those in need," possessing "an unshakable belief in where he belonged—often in harm's way"—to aid others (Carter 2014; Wilson, M. 2014). He worked with Médecins Sans Frontières, which still enjoyed a position of expert authority within the domestic debate: "That he's with Doctors Without Borders says who he is" (John Reston, quoted in McGeehan 2014). Spencer was thus the very image of the Heroic Health Worker. However, while Spencer brought this representation back to the fore, he also disrupted it. A central component of the Heroic Health Worker representation was that they were security actors, not threats. While this position of moral authority had worked to dismiss the AUT representation of threat for Brantly and Writebol, the merging of this with the dominant Hypothetical Traveler representation—and soon after Duncan—resulted in a vastly different response to Spencer. Many navigated this tension by focusing on Spencer's individual agency. Health workers were still heroic and not threatening in of themselves, but Spencer had acted dangerously. As CNN's Erin Burnett (in EB:O 2014g) summarized: "Was Dr. Craig Spencer a hero or not? Volunteering to treat Ebola patients in West Africa, but should he have known better when he came home?"

Unlike the Duncan case, where the debate raged for some time before action was taken, Spencer was met with an almost immediate practical response. Following the positive diagnosis, the (Democrat) governor of New York, Andrew Cuomo, and the (Republican) governor of New Jersey, Chris Christie, imposed a mandatory twenty-one-day quarantine for all returning health workers and West African travelers. They justified this through clear recourse to the AUT discourse:

> The fact of the matter is that I don't believe that when you are dealing with something as serious as this, that we can count on a voluntary system. . . . If anything else, the government's job is to protect the safety and the health of the citizens, and so we have taken this action. (Chris Christie, in FNS 2014c)

While the previous event had seen a diminishing of (Obama's) political authority, Spencer's diagnosis saw an effort to construct competing authorities. As Christie's statement implies, Cuomo and Christie were acting as the "protectors"—the proper sovereigns—of their populations. They were adopting a "common-sense approach," one that "the federal government wasn't taking" (Chris Christie, in Greta 2014c), and "no longer relying on the CDC standards" (Chris Christie, quoted in Santora 2014b).

This was immediately contentious. These practices—or perhaps making the AUT discourse a practical reality—seemed to have crossed a line. Media commentators brought up the impact of the extended quarantine on health workers deciding to go and help in West Africa: "single-handedly, Governors Christie and Cuomo may very well have made the situation in Africa even worse, because now fewer doctors and nurses will want to help" (Elizabeth Cohen, in TSR 2014e). Having previously shifted toward the AUT discourse and emphasized similarities, PGC proponents now reasserted their points of difference, highlighting the "economic effect" of such a policy and its "ripples" for West Africa and beyond (Rick Sacra, in AC360 2014e). HWA advocates lamented the solipsism of such a response, arguing that it demonstrated that "too many" Americans had "forgotten our brave, generous nature," "cower[ing] and whin[ing] while others suffer" (WP 2014d; see also USA Today 2014b). The White House (2014e), meanwhile, put out a statement that governors should "be guided by the science," yet remained vague in not specifically mentioning Christie or Cuomo.

While the White House refused a direct debate over the practice, one person took on the task. On the same day that these quarantine measures were put in place, Kaci Hickox arrived in Newark, New Jersey. A nurse returning from treating patients in West Africa, she was briefly recorded as having a slight fever and immediately isolated in a makeshift quarantine facility. She was kept in this quarantine despite her tests returning negative. She did not suffer through this silently. She contacted friends, one of whom spoke on her behalf to CNN (AC360 2014e; TSR 2014e). She spoke via phone with CNN's Candy Crowley from her quarantine and she wrote a letter to the *Dallas Morning News*, with excerpts quoted on television and in other newspapers:

> I sat alone in the isolation tent and thought of many colleagues who will return home to America and face the same ordeal. Will they be made to feel like criminals and prisoners? (Quoted in Newsroom 2014j; Sullivan, G. 2014a)

Hickox's arguments were twofold. In line with the broader debate, both addressed the four key sites of contestation. First, the risk to the US was not existential and therefore did not require this kind of "extreme that is really unacceptable" (SOTU 2014c). It was *West Africa* that faced the real security challenge and claims otherwise were those of irrational fear. Second, Hickox rejected the political authority Christie and Cuomo had sought to construct. This was not a case where a centralized decision was required. Indeed, for Hickox (in MTP 2014d), these decisions should be made by public health experts rather than politicians. For her supporters, Hickox was a sorely needed shake-up to the debate. She was taking a stand against the hysteria, political opportunism, and irrational extreme the Ebola response had fallen into (Layton 2014; TRMS 2014c).

Governor Christie (quoted in Rushe 2014) justified Hickox's continued quarantine by saying that she was "obviously ill" and while he was "sorry if, in any way, she was inconvenienced," he was far more concerned with "the inconvenience that could occur from having folks who are symptomatic and ill out and amongst the public." For Christie and his supporters, Hickox was insisting on "normal" civil liberties in an exceptional situation: "the public's right to remain free from Ebola outweighs your right not to be quarantined for 21 days" (Megyn Kelly, in TOF 2014e). For these speakers, Christie was exactly what they had been calling for: the sovereign who had "broken ranks" with the "political" CDC and their federal controller. His critics, meanwhile, saw him as the fearmongering, opportunistic face of the AUT discourse, playing the strongman to the fearful, irrational audience in an attempt to garner public attention, perhaps even for a run at the presidency in 2016 (Chris Matthews, in Hardball 2014d; Richard Wolffe, in PN 2014b; Sullivan, S. 2014).

Hickox, meanwhile, became the very image of the threat that an insistence on "normal politics" provided. She was "selfish," caring more about her regular "comforts" over the safety of the American people (Megyn Kelly, in TOF 2014e). Again, like Spencer, she was denied the subject-position (and moral authority) of the Heroic Health Worker. Indeed, this representation was even used against her. Kimberly Guilfoyle (in The Five 2014c) told Hickox that she should "quit crying" and instead "act that you're a nurse, you're supposed to care, you put . . . other people ahead of yourself." In the *Washington Post*, two letters to the editor used the subject-position of the audience to make the same linkage. One combined this with the authority of being a health worker herself: "I worked as a nurse for 20 years and would think it my duty to take any necessary precautions to prevent spreading a potentially fatal virus" (WP 2014e).

Hickox's challenge had mixed success. On October 27, she was flown by private plane to her home in Maine, where she was permitted to spend the rest of her mandatory quarantine at home, a change to the protocols that was expanded to all returning health workers. For Hickox, however, this was no victory. She continued to resist the quarantine, with the media avidly following her every move. News talk shows debated her actions, whether Cuomo or Christie had "caved" to federal pressure, and what this meant for the response as a whole (The Five 2014c; Kang 2014; Sullivan, G. 2014b).

In this way, the battle between Hickox and Christie (and Cuomo) provided a microcosm of the securitization of Ebola as it stood at that moment. Hickox had "the science"—and those who had aligned themselves with it—on her side, as well as the moral authority associated with her subject-position as a Heroic Health Worker who had sought to save Helpless West Africans. Yet both were challenged by the now-dominant perception that the science was uncertain (and experts untrustworthy), the audience too frightened, and the risk too great. She became "arrogant," "selfish," and even "dangerous"; an indictment of how the AUT discourse had not only dominated the debate but also reframed its competing securitizations as threatening in and of themselves. Yet the Hickox case also pointed to the fundamental instability of the AUT discourse (and its embodiment in Christie), especially in terms of its conceptualization of the exception and its legal and ethical validity. In this way, Hickox pointed to the gaps in the AUT discourse through which HWA (and PGC) approaches could be reasserted.

Together, Spencer and Hickox demonstrate the dominance of the AUT discourse established during the Thomas Eric Duncan case. They were represented as more of the hypothetical travelers made real, carrying Ebola from West Africa to American shores. Yet they were not West African Others, but white Americans. Their physical proximity to West Africa Othered them regardless. Indeed, unlike previous returning health workers (Brantly and Writebol), they were denied the subject-position of Heroic Health Worker. Yet both also challenged the AUT discourse. Hickox, in particular, directly challenged the key securitizing representations. Notably, her challenges focused on the areas of Self/Other, audience, authority, and risk as security. She revealed the instability of the AUT positions: it's denial of American benevolence, the irrationality of the audience, the illegitimacy of the Schmittian sovereign, and the lack of certainty in the emphasis on possible risk. While she did not completely destabilize the discourse, Hickox's greatest success may have been in reopening the debate.

The Midterm Elections (October–November 2014)

While Pham and Vinson recovered and Spencer and Hickox became public enemies, the midterm elections loomed. These elections, wherein all 435 seats in the House of Representatives and thirty-six of the one hundred Senate seats were contested, had been a minor focus of media coverage and political action throughout the previous events, but as November 4 drew closer, the midterms slowly eclipsed all other concerns. This did not mean a complete abandonment of these other issues and events, nor of the debates that continued around these key moments, but rather the linkage of them to the midterms and their rearticulation in accordance with the explicit partisanship that now dominated the media landscape. In other words, the midterm elections were a key event for the securitization of Ebola in terms of recontextualizing it.

In one way, the midterms simply continued the Ebola debate but provided it a more explicitly political/partisan framing. The PGC and AUT discourses were adopted and rearticulated by political hopefuls and incumbents, splitting almost evenly down partisan lines (Democrats/PGC and Republicans/AUT). Crucially, this retained the PGC shift toward the AUT representation of the (West African) threat and the (American) referent object, focusing almost exclusively (as it had during the Hickox case) on what constituted appropriate action, knowledge, and authority. New Hampshire Democratic Senator Jeanne Shaheen, for instance, argued that she was "in the camp of 'let's do what's going to work' . . . what we're hearing from medical experts and emergency response experts," while her Republican opponent, Scott Brown, insisted that "we don't need to be experts, folks, to deal with this issue" (CNN 2014a). Of course, this partisan divide was not so neat—there were Democrats advocating for travel restrictions (The Hill 2014)—but this was all subsumed into a story which "play[ed] out red news/blue news style" (Brian Stelter, in Reliable Sources 2014b). We can think of this as a formalizing of the securitization debate: the shift from a discursive contest between different definitions of the outbreak to an outright debate that was explicitly partisan. In doing so, this entrenched these positions as the two sides, narrowing the space between them and diminishing (if not erasing) the HWA discourse as a serious political alternative.

Formalizing this debate had wider impacts than simply narrowing it. In rendering the discourses explicitly partisan, the midterm elections transformed Ebola into a question about governance. David Brooks (in Brooks and Collins 2014) argued that Ebola "perfectly embod[ied a] vague sense the people running things were not quite up to the job." It was repeatedly mentioned as a core issue for voters but listed as part of a wide range of "failures of competence" of the Obama administration, sitting along scandals in Veterans Affairs and the IRS, lapses in the Secret Service, Obamacare, and even ISIS (Chris Wallace, in FNS 2014d; see also Nocera 2014; Benedetto 2014). Yet, as many commentators noted, Ebola held a special place within this list. It was perhaps even the "main thing on voters' minds" (Bump 2014b). Ebola, after all, was a threat to their security:

> When two of the four horsemen of the biblical Apocalypse come galloping out of Hell's gate—Death/Ebola and War/Islamic State—one can hardly rely on the hopers to sort things out. It's doer time. (Parker 2014)

The audience, identified by reporters through polls and interviews, was not simply frustrated with a disliked administration but "bubbling" with a "low-grade fear" that turned them away from Obama (Maggie Haberman, in CNN 2014b; see also Chen 2014; Fisher 2014).

The results of the midterms seemed to confirm this. Republicans not only took control of the Senate but achieved the largest Senate gain (for either Republicans or Democrats) since 1980. In the House of Representatives, they expanded their majority by thirteen seats: the largest majority they had enjoyed since the Great Depression. Ultimately, the midterms, as Carter Eskew (2014) evocatively described it, demonstrated that "the country wants its daddy": the "tough, stern ruler of the house" to protect them from threats like ISIS and Ebola.

Following this resounding Republican victory and the linking of the AUT understanding of Ebola's threat to it, two responses can be observed in those of opposing leanings. The first is an increased shift toward the AUT approach. The day after the midterms, Obama requested an additional $6.18 billion in "emergency appropriations" for Ebola. In his letter to the Speaker, he outlined that his "foremost priority is to protect the health and safety of Americans" and "prevent additional cases at home" (Obama

2014j). Within the actual funding request, there was also a significant portion directed at domestic preparedness efforts, including Ebola treatment units. The majority, however, was for efforts in West Africa in quelling the outbreak, so this was not a complete abandonment of the referent object and threat of the PGC discourse but rather yet another qualification of its emphasis to align with the dominant AUT approach.

The second, and perhaps most important, response was a powerful reiteration of the Fearbola discourse. The midterms were presented here not as a marker of any objective problem, whether in the immediate Ebola response or the Obama presidency, but instead as a testament to Republicans' manipulation of fear for political gain. They had run on a platform of "pure negativity" (NYT 2014e), exploiting the audience's wider "anxiety about an increasingly dangerous world" (Wittle and Fifield 2014) through focusing on "Ebola in the scariest, most non-factual ways" (Andrea Mitchell, in MSNBC 2014). Others ascribed the blame to the media, whose "breathless pursuit of [Ebola] carriers in this country" created the fears Republicans exploited (Wickham 2014b). In other words, while the AUT discourse remained (and was recognized as) dominant, it was reproduced less as a reflection of reality than as an act of opportunistic politics or of Fearbola. This challenge was effective, both in encouraging some Republicans to reiterate their audience-driven relationship with the politics of fear (Rubin 2014b) and, more crucially, in recontextualizing the debate.

The midterms were reframed as the moment wherein the securitization of Ebola finally had political repercussions. The securitization of Ebola thus moved from a debate on the reality of Ebola's security dimension to one of what this meant politically:

> What scares you about Ebola? What scares me is not that I might get infected here in New York City. The odds of that are infinitesimal, tiny. What does scare me, though, are the mass of contradictory responses, from local, state, and federal officials. What scares me are the politics of Ebola. (Brian Stelter, in Reliable Sources 2014b)

This took two broad forms. The first was a concern with the effects of securitization, namely the politics of fear on US society. Commentators highlighted the point that, as fear took hold, neither Republicans nor "the people" accorded much respect to medical expertise (Blake 2014; Bruni 2014; Perez-Pena 2014; Somin 2014). The second form of political recontextualization was a more reflexive consideration of what precisely was at play in securitizing Ebola. Angelique Kidjo (2014), for instance, drew attention to the deeply racialized narratives that underpinned the fears surrounding Ebola, namely the "fears and fantasies of Africa as the Heart of Darkness." Even the representation of "West African Fragility," central to each of the discourses and their understanding of causation in the outbreak, was challenged here. Karen Attiah (2014), for instance, argued that West Africans were not "just sitting around waiting to be saved by the United States," but instead had saved themselves while the US was lost in its own "fear, hysteria, quarantines and stigmatization."

Ultimately, the midterms provided a moment of reflexivity, a vantage point from which the political construction of Ebola as a security issue could be seriously considered. The elections encouraged the formalizing of the PGC/AUT debate, reframing each discourse in partisan terms and linking their key representations to broader contextual discourses of governance and politics. In doing so, however, both discourses were destabilized. The dominance of the AUT approach—especially its construction of the audience—was affirmed, but its contingency was also revealed. Again, this centralized around four key areas: the Othering of West Africa to the point of threat, the terrified audience, the need for a "strong" sovereign and the diminishing of experts, and the understanding of security and exception via risk. Yet these were now represented as partisan talking points and explored, questioned, and challenged on this basis. In following these fraying threads, persistent members of the media and oppositional politicians found no solid grounding, destabilizing the discourses premised on them.

Silence, Withdrawal, and Desecuritization (November 2014–February 2015)

The midterms ultimately provided the beginning of the end for the securitization of Ebola. Attention to the disease dropped dramatically. Some of this, particularly the latter drop in focus, is attributable to the outbreak itself slowly coming under control and the lack of US-specific events. Yet November cannot be completely explained this way. A number of notable events occurred during this month—including the evacuation and death of Dr. Martin Salia between November 14 and 17—and the outbreak continued to threaten West Africa (even appearing in Mali). Yet Ebola still slid from the headlines, and this happened at a pace striking enough without even considering the change in substance that accompanied it.

Focusing on the latter, however, demonstrates that Ebola was not simply dropped as a concern but reframed as a past one. The threat of Ebola, in other words, was over. Ebola was now "this summer's emergency" (CFA 2014c, 15). In a particularly unambiguous framing, MSNBC's Chris Hayes (in All In 2014b) announced that November 11 was "VE day, that's 'victory over Ebola' day." Even the flurry of new bills introduced into Congress, largely pertaining to the prohibition of flights and the issuance of visas[5], was framed with a shifting threat perception: "it's not just Ebola I'm worried about . . . it is what is coming" (Kelly 2014). The significance of this temporal framing lies in its corresponding shift of focus. Current and future events were no longer the central concern. Perhaps the most striking demonstration of this was the coverage (or lack thereof) of Dr. Salia. Evacuated to the US on November 15 for treatment, he died on November 17, becoming the second person to die from Ebola on American soil. Despite this, he was covered largely only in periodic updates, if covered at all. USA Today, for instance, did not mention him.

Instead, the coverage turned to what the lessons from Ebola should be. It became, in other words, a debate over "the Ebola story" (Krugman 2014). The high-profile American cases were revisited: Nina Pham, Amber Joy Vinson, and Craig Spencer. Crucially, this coverage overwhelmingly took the form of reaffirming their subject-positioning as Heroic Health Workers. Vinson and Pham, for instance, were labeled "heroes," going "into a potentially deadly situation" without hesitation "because it is their job" (John Berman and Christine Romans, in Early Start 2014e). Spencer's case was rewritten, with wider conclusions drawn about the domestic response: "nobody got sick while he was in New York," noted CNN's Elizabeth Cohen (in Newsroom 2014k), "in other words, the health authorities were right."

This reformation of health workers was a piece of a wider representation of "the Ebola story" as one of the PGC discourse's (and its advocates', namely the Obama administration and CDC Director Frieden) validation. The possible—the basis for the AUT's construction of threat—had not happened. The production of knowledge from uncertainty was not a "common sense" consideration of the worst-case scenario, but a complete disregard of medical expertise. Experts had "said all along" that it was hard to get Ebola, and "time has shown us" that they got it right (Elizabeth Cohen, in TSR 201fj; see also Krugman 2014). The PGC/AUT debate, accordingly, was over. The PGC approach was validated, while the AUT discourse became

Fearbola, the irrational, emotive, and deeply political construction worthy only of mockery, disgust, and embarrassment.

The problem with this, of course, was that while the public debate shifted to the past, the actual outbreak in West Africa continued very much in the present. This was a particular concern of HWA proponents, who resurfaced to occupy this newly vacated space in covering the outbreak (notably in the *New York Times* and the *Washington Post*), and the Obama administration. While their focus differed slightly, both were concerned that, as the explicitly solipsistic forms of securitization lessened their hold on the public's imagination, the US public discussion was not moving toward a "better" securitization but complete desecuritization. Médecins Sans Frontières's Dr. Joanne Liu (quoted in Gladstone 2014) labeled this the prospect of a "double failure": "a response that was slow to begin with and is ill-adapted at the end." Reporters, commentators, politicians, and even the UN's secretary-general, Ban Ki-Moon (2014), engaged in constant "reminders" that the outbreak was not over, adding "another concern . . . to the list: declaring 'mission accomplished' too soon." Such concerns were not without merit. By December, it was widely accepted that Ebola was no longer a topic of public concern (Sargent 2014). Meanwhile, Obama's post-midterm request for $6.18 billion still required congressional approval, and it was bundled within a wider spending bill that increased the chance of it being shortchanged for other priorities.

The Obama administration's response was to reiterate the continued threat to the US. Obama himself engaged in this reiteration during a trip to the National Institutes of Health on December 2:

> I realize that here in the United States, some of the attention has shifted away recently—that's sort of how our attention spans work sometimes. Ebola is not leading the news right now. But I wanted to come here because, every day, we're focused on keeping the American people safe. . . . [And] the fight is not even close to being over. As long as this case continues to rage in West Africa, we could continue to see isolated cases here in America. (Obama 2014k)

The emergency funding request was approved, with Congress appropriating $5.4 billion for the continued response and longer-term "preparedness." More than two-thirds of this was allocated for international efforts (with the bulk of it going to the lead agency, USAID), with $1.1 billion focused toward domestic preparedness. Considering Congress's reticence to fund Obama's policies, this appropriation—the largest ever committed to a single health crisis—was still viewed by many as a success and a clear "emergency measure" (Nakamura 2014b; Parker and Weisman 2014; WP 2014f).

For some, however, this moment of "success" risked providing a neat conclusion to a security issue that was neither neat nor concluded. Suggestions that US troops would be brought home sparked concerns that the US was abandoning West Africa right when the outbreak could be completely extinguished. This was acted on by Sen. Chris Coons (2015), who wrote to Defense Secretary Hagel in January 2015 that "the fight against Ebola is far from over," and a continued US response was vital. The problem, as Coons outlined, was that the continued emergency response was vital, but how do you ensure this without falling into the Schmittian politics that had skewed it previously?

Obama answered this by claiming success. In February 2015, he provided an update on the "Ebola fight," where he explicitly stated that the strategy was "transitioning" to a more public-health-oriented one and all but one hundred of the 2,400 US troops in West Africa would return by April 30. That said, however, it remained crucial to "get . . . to zero" because "as long as there is even one case of Ebola that's active out there, risks still exist" (Obama 2015). This was, ultimately, a reiteration of the PGC discourse within the aftermath of the AUT approach; a careful reminder that while the US was acting entirely for its own safety (repeatedly asserting "this is not charity"), it needed to take a wider definition of its self-interest:

> And in the 21st century, we cannot build moats around our countries. There are no drawbridges to be pulled up. We shouldn't try. What we should do is instead make sure everybody has basic health systems—from hospitals to disease detectives to better laboratory networks—all of which allows us to get early warnings against outbreaks of diseases. (Obama 2015)

Obama's (2015) speech, as some noted, reflected his own vindication after the long and grueling fight over the Ebola narrative, noting the "weeks in which all too often we heard science being ignored and sensationalism." Yet this was not simply an "I told you so" (Condon 2015). It was also an effort to neatly conclude the securitization of Ebola, to move away from the security framing to one of public health and development.

Ultimately, Obama did successfully close the securitization process. Crucially, he did so in a way that enabled him to persist with measures while closing off the potential for more extreme forms. Of course, this would not have been possible if a process of desecuritization (through neglect) had not already taken place. Indeed, it could easily be asserted that the securitization of Ebola ended after the midterm elections. It is worth ending here, however, because Obama's careful closure of the formal discussion speaks to where exactly the process had come. It speaks to the institutional power a government holds once the audience's attentions have (ostensibly) shifted and how even that power is qualified by the discursive reality that had been produced.

Conclusion

This chapter focused on the contested process of securitization over the Ebola outbreak. It traced the contestation and alignment between the four basic discourses outlined in the previous chapter, highlighting the nuanced evolutions, the points of insurmountable difference, and the way both of these came together to form the US's Ebola response. It revealed four key sites of contestation: the reconstruction of the Self/Other relationship and its linkages to threat and referent, the representation of the accepting audience, the subject-positions of moral, political, and expert authority, and security's meaning and logic. It is at each of these sites that particular discourses both dominated and were diminished at particular times. It is within these spaces that the process of securitization truly shifted and evolved.

We could perhaps summarize this process through two speeches by President Obama: his September 16 speech to the CDC and his final update on February 11. In the former, he outlined the devastating effects the outbreak was having on West Africa, focusing on the "absolutely gut-wrenching" stories he had heard from West Africa (Obama 2014b). "These men and women and children are just sitting, waiting to die, right now," he noted. Nearly six months later, he framed his government's response to the outbreak differently: "this is not charity" (Obama 2015). Self-interest was not absent in that early speech, nor was the plight of the West African entirely missing in the latter one. But the weighting had changed. The meaning had changed. Ultimately, the underlying discourse had changed.

Yet while the ending offers a neat way of summarizing this process, it is important not to dismiss the rest of this process as simply that: the process leading to this point. The securitization of Ebola was an ongoing reality, one that shifted and evolved as new events needed to be adapted to. Each moment, each event, and each dynamic at play is important. Kent Brantly, Nancy Writebol, and the media coverage of them—expanding the ethical boundaries of the referent object but still grounded in American risk—mattered for when and how the Obama administration finally responded. The debate over Obama's response mattered for Thomas Eric Duncan, Nina Pham, and Amber Joy Vinson, as the former became evidence of the possible West African threat and the latter two victims of Obama's certainty. This denial of certainty and the authority that proclaimed it certainly mattered for Craig Spencer and Kaci Hickox, who found themselves vilified and even confined on the basis that they risked an American pandemic. And all of this mattered for the midterm elections, where Republicans formally presented themselves as the defenders of the terrified public and swept to victory on the claim that they would enact the common sense exception. Each of these points was a decisive moment in the securitization of Ebola, but the securitization of Ebola was also decisive in defining, responding to, and ultimately forming each event.

5 Securitizing beyond Ebola

Introduction

This book started with two questions: How was Ebola securitized and what role did contestation play in this response? Answers are apparent in the previous chapters, but here I focus on them explicitly, bringing the detail together into the larger findings of this analysis. I start with the specific, outlining the four key findings from the Ebola case. The first three of these four correspond to the four key sites of contestation outlined in the previous chapter. First, all the securitizing discourses were ultimately premised on a (re)construction of the Self/Other, though they differed on the temporal and ethical meaning they ascribed to this relationship. Second, the audience and authority were key. Constructions of the former gave meaning to the latter, which split into three different forms (political, expert, and moral). Third, uncertainty—and the construction of threat through risk—was prime. Speculating about remote possibilities allowed for extreme scenarios to be presented, and they could not be entirely dismissed. Claiming certainty, moreover, was dangerous: it opened actors to the representation of being too cavalier about the possible threat. The final of the four findings takes these claims and considers the broader political significance of them: how these discourses and the key sites of contestation shaped the US's response to Ebola. While the previous chapter outlined this in detail, here I focus on the bigger picture. Ultimately, this response was far too late, with US involvement seemingly waiting for the distant tragedy of Ebola to finally manifest as a potential national security threat. It also—despite some practices that did center West Africans—tended to focus on short-term containment. Perhaps most problematically, this emphasis on containment combined with the tendency toward Othering, the fearful American Self, and the logic of risk to reinscribe the neglect of Ebola, defined here as an absence of care to those suffering and the conditions that led to it.

I then consider what this study of the US response to Ebola provides to the wider study of securitization and contemporary security in general. The first two chapters of this book (and the first half of this chapter) were dedicated to what securitization theory brings to our understanding of this response, but what of the reverse? This book has offered a detailed examination of domestic-level securitization and the role of contestation within it. What does this case contribute to wider, contemporary debates surrounding securitization? While this book provides numerous minor contributions, I focus here on the more substantive insights. First, I reiterate the importance of context for securitization but again the need to consider context as a malleable, contested construction. Securitization ultimately borrows from and fits within wider social debates: the nature of the Self, the Other, the threat of disease, and so on. Second, I explore how the Ebola case testifies to the multiplicity of security's meaning and logic. Security remains sedimented in a solipsistic and externalized understanding of threat, yet this "thickness" is never completely insurmountable. I also connect the issues of authority and knowledge to the underpinning logic of security: exceptionalism. The Ebola case, as I argue, attests to the potentiality of exceptionalism and the need to consider it in more detail. It ultimately offers a window into how global health can be dominated by claims to the Schmittian exception (the America Under Threat [AUT] discourse) but can also be challenged and reformulated without necessarily denying the exceptional nature of disease outbreaks. And finally, this chapter returns to the foundational idea of securitization as a political process. Even in its most extreme, Schmittian forms, securitization is always entwined with the messy realm of normal politics, infused with the mundane debates over domestic matters and occupied by myriad actors that range from the sovereign to a member of the audience writing to the editor. Securitization is thus not a single elite speech act but rather an evolving and contested process of meaning production.

The US Securitization of Ebola

The previous chapters together provided an exploration of the US securitization of Ebola: both how it was variously understood as a security threat (chapter three) and how these securitizing discourses interacted to form the process of securitization that occurred between July 2014 to February 2015 (chapter four). Across these chapters, several key findings become evident. There are points of commonality between the securitizing discourses that became central to the wider construction of the outbreak as a security concern. There are also particularly vital points of difference, which became central in enabling the dominance of some discourses and the marginalization of others, having crucial impacts on the response. Here, I outline four empirical insights—four key components of the US securitization of Ebola—which both allow a firm conclusion to the case study and provide insights of theoretical significance for the discussion on securitization theory.

The Self/Other Relationship and Its Formulation as Friend/Enemy

Each of the securitizing discourses relied on a Self/Other foundation. The Self, in all cases, was the US as the Indispensable Nation: advanced, powerful, and moral. The world—and West Africa in particular—could not survive without its intervention. The Other, meanwhile, was the "inferior" West African: backward, powerless, and barbaric. The Ebola outbreak was directly linked to this, presented as a consequence of "West African Fragility." The commonality of these representations, and their clear construction through differentiation of the Other, speaks to the centrality of the Self/Other relationship (and identity) to securitizing discourses. This, of course, is not a new finding for either securitizing or disease discourses (Hansen 2006; Wald 2008), but it provides a foundation for the more striking insight: contestation over the Other as enemy.

The Self/Other relationship, despite being common, was a site of significant contestation. For the AUT discourse, the West African was a source of threat. They were inherently—and eternally—inferior as ignorant, superstitious, and diseased. For the Potential Global Catastrophe (PGC) discourse, West Africans were also the inferior Other, but this had a crucial temporal element: "Africa needing" against "Africa rising" (Gerson 2014a). West Africa was understood as a site between the two, with its "fledgling democracies" (CFA 2014a, 22) making "progress . . . in overcoming conflict and improving economic development" (CFA 2014b, 8) but also facing "challenges" from its own inadequacies (Rice 2014). Meanwhile, for Helpless West Africa (HWA) advocates, West Africa's inferiority again took a different form. In emphasizing the extreme level of insecurity, HWA proponents stripped the agency from their representation of West Africa, leaving them as passive victims in need of (American) salvation. Each of these was a construction of the inferior Other against the superior Self; the inferiority of West Africa gave the US's indispensability meaning, but the nature of American superiority was also integral to understanding just how West Africa was supposed to have failed.

Similarly, it is in the Self/Other relationship that the significance of these different Others can be observed. Simply put, it outlined an ethical standing, a position to take on West Africa's suffering. The AUT and PGC discourses ultimately ascribed a level of blame to West Africa and its people. AUT advocates used their understanding to present the Self as endangered by the Other. PGC proponents made a similar claim but presented saving the Other (stopping it from disintegrating) as saving the Self. As Rep. Christopher Smith (in CFA 2014b, 8) summarized, "Ebola has demonstrated that our neighbor's problems can soon become our problems." The HWA approach, however, drastically altered this Self/Other dynamic. Rather than a threat to the Self, the Other was the referent object. Even more strikingly, it was precisely their Otherness that rendered them such (and, in conjunction, rendered the Self as safe). Othering, rather than a way of dismissing moral obligation, was employed to produce it.

This is, in essence, an articulation not simply of Self/Other but of friend/enemy. In fact, it points to the differences between the two. The Self/Other dynamic does not necessarily conform to the antagonistic relationship noted by Schmitt (and the Copenhagen School formulation of securitization theory). The HWA discourse, after all, testifies to this. While it reiterated the Othering of West Africa through the West African Fragility representation, it did not construct this Other as the "enemy" or source of threat. Rather, it constructed the Other as a figure worthy of sympathy, aid, and, most importantly, protection. Within the Schmittian formulation that underpins securitization theory, this renders the West African Other the "friend": the referent to protect. In doing so, it provided a constant challenge to the other securitizing discourses. In some isolated cases, this was successful. The debate over using experimental treatments, for instance, became subsumed into a consideration of whose lives were worth exceptional intervention and why West Africa was denied this position. The plight of the Other could not be entirely dismissed.

Yet the plight of the Other also could not be entirely considered as, after all, it diminished the emphasis on the Self. Crucially, it undermined the ethical viability of such a priority, diluting the enemy against which the threat to the friend/Self could be defined. Accordingly, while it enjoyed some minor successes, for the most part this attempt to reproduce the Other as friend left the HWA discourse unstable. Some AUT proponents explicitly challenged it, reasserting the moral primacy of the Self against the danger it faced, thus presenting the HWA—and any PGC proponents aligning with it—as ignoring "us" for "them" (Keith Ablow, quoted in Wemple 2014a). Others simply ignored it, but their reproductions of the Other as enemy diminished the HWA approach regardless. The friend/enemy distinction was thus a key site of contention—with the AUT discourse stabilizing at the cost of the HWA approach—despite its Self/Other foundation being strikingly common otherwise.

It is also worth highlighting the role of contextual discourses in this production of the friend/enemy distinction. The positioning of the West African Other as a friend aligns with discourses of disease as a humanitarian issue, particularly in its challenge to conceptions of disease as a security threat to the Self (see Harman and Wenham 2018). Yet the contesting claims of West Africa as the enemy Other were also contextual, drawing on the long-running Dark Continent discourse. Africa still invokes a particular imaginary within the US public context, one that is employed, reiterated, and evolved by actors in cases like this. This is never inevitable, as the HWA and even the PGC discourses suggest, but this history provides its modern reiterations a weight that is difficult to contest. Moreover, there are few public counternarratives about (West) Africa. Accordingly, the idea of West Africa as a threat via a disease outbreak fit an already entrenched reality of Africa as a "dirty and diseased place" (Seay and Dionne 2014).

The Centrality of the Audience and Authority

Another crucial site of commonality between the securitizing discourses— and, perhaps just as importantly, the Fearbola counterdiscourse—was the centrality of the audience. Each speaker sought to claim that they spoke on behalf of the American people, presenting their understanding of the outbreak and its response in line with what the people wanted, felt, or needed. This was the case even when actors were immediately speaking to another audience, such as the president, members of the administration (including the CDC director), or political opponents:

> This should be a very top priority of the White House, the political leadership of the Nation. We know the career people, what they are going to do, but [what] of the White House? Because the American people deserve to know what their government leadership is doing to prevent the spread of this epidemic and keep the country safe. (Frank Wolf, in CFA 2014a, 7)

What precisely was meant by "the American people" however, was deeply contested. Contestation reigned over each and every point of evidence offered to illustrate this audience: opinion polls provided different numbers, anecdotes could always be matched with an opposing anecdote, who was allowed to speak as the audience in the media was carefully curated, and even the midterm results could be qualified by noting that the turnout was quite low and Republicans worried about Ebola may have been more incited to vote than those thinking differently (see Bump 2014b). It could easily be argued that actors actually spoke to different audiences within the wider American people (AUT proponents to Republican voters, for instance), yet they always sought to present this as the real American people and themselves as speaking on behalf of this uniform body. The audience, in other words, was not truly important as a uniform, objective entity that actors fought over but instead was vital as a site of legitimation.

Speakers used these constructions of the audience to legitimate their positions and, crucially, themselves. AUT proponents were simply voicing the people's fears, asking the questions they wanted to ask, and looking to minimize the ostensible danger they faced. PGC proponents, in contrast, presented themselves as upholding the higher values of the American people: a refusal to "give in" to fear, a reverence for science, and a willingness to shoulder global burdens (Obama 2014c; 2014i). And the Fearbola counterdiscourse, which was frequently employed by the HWA discourse on this front, presented itself as the truth-teller: it mocked audience irrationality, criticized elites for manipulating them, and suggested that a better, more rational audience was possible. In doing so, it ultimately made an appeal to those who would be in the audience to eschew the fearmongering representation offered by the others and take instead the more self-reflexive position in line with its own approach. Accordingly, the contestation over who and what the audience (or the American people) were was rather one of who could speak/act and how.

This directly informed contests around speaker and actor authority. Authority concerns the precise power the speaker holds: how and why it can speak, act, and be heard/adhered to. It enables particular speech and action, and it restrains others. In the first chapter, I borrowed from Holger Stritzel (2014, 50–51) the idea of "processes of authorization," where authority is constructed, accepted, reiterated, challenged, debated, and sometimes completely dismissed. As the previous chapter demonstrated in detail, this process of authorization was key to discursive (in)stability. Undermining particular forms of authority destabilized the PGC discourse, namely its key representations of certainty, appropriate response, and the exception. Producing authority and reaffirming it against the diminishment of others heightened AUT dominance, particularly opening the necessary space in which the possible threat could be constructed. The process of authorization, in other words, was a key site of contestation and it was one that was exceedingly important for the process of securitization that occurred.

Differing types of authority were evident in this process: political, moral, and medical/expert. Each was constructed through the production of a speaker-audience relationship, but the precise nature of this relationship varied. Political authority was essentially the speaker-audience relationship discussed above: the speaker as speaking/acting on behalf of the audience (the people). In addition to being the speaker, however, political authority was also crucially entwined with the subject-position of the sovereign. Political authorities were the protectors of the people, the upholder of the fundamental social contract as enshrined contextually within the US Constitution, and the deciders of the exception. Moral authority was not predicated on the positioning of an actor as acting on behalf of an audience. Rather, they were presented as embodying the American ideal, someone who ultimately represented the best of the American audience. Accordingly, they did not speak for the audience, but they represented its better nature: its values, its ethical priorities, and its best attributes (rationality, humanitarianism, and capability). And medical/expert authority concerned the important question of who could provide knowledge. If political authority denotes one who can speak/act on the audience's behalf, the expert authority is one that the audience (and the political authority) can (or should) listen to. In this sense, the speaker-audience relationship was one of trust and guidance. The very (re)production of the expert subject-position involves a construction of them as trustworthy and knowledgeable in a way that laypersons lack. The two are crucial: experts are widely understood as those with exclusive knowledge who can neutrally apply said knowledge to problems. Their authority relies on these twin components of neutrality and expertise.

By adopting a position of authority, speakers could challenge other positions of authority and the discourse of security they proposed. The moral authority of the Heroic Health Worker was used to challenge claims to political authority, namely those of AUT proponents. This was apparent in the immediate rejection of the AUT production of Kent Brantly and Nancy Writebol as threats. Brantly and Writebol's positioning as "inspiring role models" and "serv[ing] on the front lines" quickly reframed those suggesting that they be left to treatment in Liberia as unethical, irrational, and even unpatriotic (Siegel 2014; WP 2014a). Yet the triumph of the moral authority over the political one was never certain, as demonstrated aptly by Kaci Hickox. Hickox explicitly used her position as a moral authority in her public battle against Chris Christie (SOTU 2014c). Yet Christie responded in kind, presenting his position as political authority as paramount and questioning Hickox's moral authority (FNS 2014c). Political authority was also employed to challenge expert authority, namely in the notion of acting in "common sense" against the "confusing and incoherent" "expertise" offered (Scott Brown, in CNN 2014a). These concerted efforts to diminish expert authority, however, were largely due to the success of experts in diminishing claims to political authority, particularly in August and September against travel bans. Even at its height, the notion that political authority could simply overturn expertise was contestable: "if you were president, and NIH or the CDC were saying, hey, you know, this will only make it worse, a travel ban, a flight ban, will only make it worse, what we have in place is better, you would overrule the doctors and the experts?" (Candy Crowley, in SOTU 2014b).

These various claims to authority were not deconstructed just by the challenge itself, however. Opponents directly attacked the foundations of each construction of authority, seeking to reveal a disjuncture between an actor's claim to authority and the authority itself. Political authority relied on the positioning of the speaker as acting as the sovereign on behalf of the audience. Contestation, accordingly, revolved around presenting political authorities—namely the institutionalized authority of the president—as misaligned with the audience, acting on their own (political) behalf, and abrogating their sovereign power to decide. Opponents frequently claimed this while simultaneously representing themselves as the proper authority figure. Expert authority, meanwhile, was challenged on the basis that they had been politicized, their required neutrality and expertise missing: "the doctors and the experts that are saying this are working for the administration and repeating the administration talking points" (Ted Cruz, in SOTU 2014b). Moral authority was primarily constructed through the Heroic Health Worker representation: a self-sacrificing and rational humanitarian actor saving the Other at great cost to the Self. Kaci Hickox provides the clearest case of this being disputed. She was "selfish" and "arrogant" in prioritizing her own "comfort" over the protection of other Americans. Accordingly, her claims to the greater harm being produced by the quarantine policy, as well as her appeal to upholding civil liberties, could be dismissed without being labeled immoral.

There were also practical manifestations of this contestation. Competing claims to audience and authority grounded contradictory policies. The New York/New Jersey implementation of mandatory quarantine for returning health workers, for instance, was fundamentally a rebuke of White House policy, dismissing their insistence that current measures—airport screenings, testing, and contact tracing—were sufficient. Crucially, this was presented as a fulfillment of "the government's job . . . to protect the safety and health of our citizens," a job the federal government was explicitly claimed to be ignoring (Chris Christie, in FNS 2014c). It was also represented as a common sense choice against incoherent and politicized expertise. The White House and Obama's responses, meanwhile, were to reiterate their position and denigrate this practice as that of irrational or manipulative actors, not the demands of the rational, brave, and benevolent audience (see Obama 2014h, 2014i, 2014k). In essence, the representation of audience and authority were central to policies that were explicitly at odds.

Ultimately, speaker authority (and the process of authorization) became crucial to the contest over which securitizing discourse offered the truth on the Ebola outbreak and its threat. It underpinned who could speak, who should be listened to, who could be dismissed, and on what grounds all of this could occur. Again, this was centered on the audience, but not any objective audience. This was a careful construction of a speaker-audience relationship, one that placed members of the public into a subject-position they could speak from (and they did, to varied effects) but was ultimately more focused on producing a position of power, of validity, and of authority that securitizing actors could speak from.

The Primacy of Risk Logics in Defining Security

The third, but perhaps most crucial, finding from analyzing the US securitization of Ebola concerns the role of risk logics in defining security. The Copenhagen School, as the first chapter explained, defines security according to the Schmittian logic of exceptionalism: it concerns a direct and imminent threat to one's existence, necessitating the suspension of normal politics. Yet two of the key securitizing discourses evident during the US process of securitizing Ebola did not entirely conform to this logic: the AUT discourse focused on a hypothetical danger in the future and the PGC discourse insisted on an indirect and possible threat. Both of these relied, at least partially, on a logic of risk to define security. The significance of this finding goes beyond what it informs us about this particular case. It ultimately disputes a core assumption of the original Copenhagen School's approach to security, and it demands a reconsideration of how we understand exceptionalism as a political phenomenon.

Here, I refer to risk in the same manner as many others employing it in relation to securitization. Olaf Corry (2012, 235) describes it as "oriented towards the conditions of possibility or constitutive causes of harm, a kind of 'second-order' security politics that promotes long-term precautionary governance." Claudia Aradau, Luis Lobo-Guerrero, and Rens van Munster (2007, 149) similarly describe risk as implying "a specific relation to the future, a relation that requires a monitoring of the future, an attempt to calculate what the future can offer, and a need to control and minimize its potentially harmful effects." Ultimately, we can understand risk through three key tenets: risk is future-oriented and thus uncertain; risk is concerned with perpetual vulnerability, emphasizing conditional, indirect causes of harm; and risk is ultimately concerned with danger management, shifting from "a politics of emergency and exceptionality [to] a politics of permanence and long-termism" (Corry 2012, 245). Many in this area contrast this logic of risk against the logic of security within securitization theory. Risk is, as Aradau et al. (2008, 149) note, often viewed as the "more mundane concept": temporally, causally, and practically stretched from the imminent, existential, and exceptional (in the Schmittian sense) threat of security. Indeed, the contrast is viewed by some—notably Wæver (2011,

474)—as so stark as to necessitate their complete separation: "risk is risk, and securitization is securitization."

The AUT and PGC discourses both constructed their central dangers in line with this understanding of risk. Both defined the threat as the possibility of harm, speculating on the future of the outbreak rather than its present danger. They also understood the US as vulnerable, observing this as key to the danger they faced, and thus emphasized the need for preparedness. From this general commonality, however, they diverged. The AUT discourse understood the future threat through speculation from uncertainty; danger was thus hypothetical but direct. In the face of this existential (but hypothetical) danger, vulnerability, whether through the Hypothetical Traveler or the lack of emergency response, was unacceptable. Ted Cruz (2014a) aptly captured this construction of risk, asking: "what if, God forbid, we saw 8,000 [patients], as in West Africa? . . . We shouldn't risk finding out what that answer might be." For the PGC approach, enough certainty existed that the probability of danger could be calculated or, at the very least, speculated on from this knowledge basis. The danger for these speakers was thus largely indirect—economic, political, or circulatory—and vulnerability to the direct threat could be managed. As Obama (2014c) outlined in his UN speech:

> If this epidemic is not stopped, this disease could cause a humanitarian catastrophe across the region. And in an era where regional crises can quickly become global threats, stopping Ebola is in the interest of all of us.

This more probable, indirect danger required emergency action, but did not require the invocation of a dramatic domestic exception. In essence, the debate between these two positions (which, as the previous chapter demonstrated, was core to the overarching process of securitization) was one of what kind of risk underpinned the claim to security and what kind of exception it demanded.

Does this mean then that Wæver is correct in his separation of risk and securitization, with this instead a debate about risk rather than security? Such a claim would miss two important points. Firstly, despite focusing on a future and indirect threat in need of management, Obama (2014b, 2014c; in MTP 2014b) still openly declared this a "national security" problem. Security remained the label under which these discussions occurred, with risk proposed as a variant of it. Secondly, but perhaps more importantly, the traditional logic of security still pervaded this discussion. The

PGC discourse, for instance, frequently aligned itself with constructions of more immediate, existential danger, specifically the HWA understanding of threat in its early formulations ("right now, the world still has an opportunity to save countless lives") and the AUT approach to possible existential threat in later ones ("this is not charity; we do this because the world is interconnected"). The merging of risk and security logics, however, is especially apparent in the AUT discourse. The AUT approach did produce a hypothetical future danger, yet it was also an existential danger: it was a direct threat to the lives and wellbeing of Americans. Moreover, it demanded the kind of exceptionalism that the Copenhagen School and others of a Schmittian focus identify as central to security: an alteration to normal routines and policies, including the violation of civil liberties. AUT proponents were not seeking to manage the risk, seeing this as an "intolerable" state of vulnerability, but sought to eliminate it entirely (Cruz 2014a). In other words, while we can pinpoint the basic logic of risk underwriting these constructions, it is impossible to entirely extract it from that of security.

Ultimately, the Ebola case affirms risk as a logic of exceptionalism. More specifically, it affirms that exceptionalism must be read as a larger spectrum of political possibility, as outlined in the first chapter. This will be discussed in more detail later in this chapter, when we consider what this case tells us about securitization theory, but for now, it is worth simply emphasizing the significance of this finding. We cannot understand the US securitization of Ebola without understanding securitization in terms of multiple security logics. Attempts to split these logics—Wæver's (2011, 474) "risk is risk, and securitization is securitization" and Corry's (2012) separate framework of "riskification," for instance—would only fragment our analysis of the Ebola response and leave us with detrimental gaps in our understanding. We would either have to strip the risk or the security from analysis or provide a direct comparison of riskifying and securitizing discourse that misses both the interplay between them and the fact that risk and security frequently merged into one claim to danger. Within securitization theory, this is a somewhat contentious position, but this analysis demonstrates it a necessary one.

Multiple Discourses, One Response

So far, this discussion has largely focused on the internal dynamics of the American securitization of Ebola and the interplay between them. These findings offer important insights into how and why the securitization of Ebola progressed and evolved as it did. Yet there remains one final step in this analysis: one to the bigger picture. What does all this tell us about the US response to Ebola? How did the securitization of Ebola—the contested process that it was—ultimately shape the response in West Africa and in the US? After all, besides the domestic actions of state governors, this was still one response: that of the Obama administration. The Obama administration sent the US military to aid in West Africa, refused travel and trade restrictions, and implemented enhanced airport screenings. The Department of State's USAID enacted their disaster assistance response teams to aid the international response. The CDC provided guidelines, training, and aid to both West Africa and affected locations (hospitals) in the US. The previous chapter demonstrated in detail how their positions and actions were made possible (and impossible) by the shifting boundaries of Ebola's securitization. Let us now examine this with a wider focus, considering the response as a whole.

Firstly, the response was late. The Obama administration claimed that they had been involved since March 2014, when the CDC first sent staff to the affected nations (White House 2014b, 2014c). Yet the CDC itself later described this as a "very limited" response, with few staff on the ground, until the activation of its Emergency Operations Center on July 9 (Dahl et al. 2016, 12). Meanwhile, the response at this point was limited to the CDC and USAID, with the Department of Defense only establishing a task force in August and the military becoming involved in September (JCOA 2016, 5). This delay detrimentally impacted the response. For instance, while the military focused on building Ebola treatment units to manage the increasing caseload, many of them were not built in time to be used (JCOA 2016, 49). Under the CDC's expanded guidance, Liberia only established an incident management system in late July, which proved vital for Liberia's response (Dahl et al. 2016, 16).

Part of this delay is due to the nature of the outbreak and international response. It was mistakenly believed (especially by the WHO) that the outbreak had been contained in May 2014. June, however, saw cases rise again, with exponential growth in July. Yet another part is due to heightened public attention during this period. An evaluation by members of the CDC, for instance, notes "the world's attention" as core to why "considerable additional staff were deployed" in late July and early August (Dahl et al.

2016, 16). The timing of this is clear: this was the point at which securitization was occurring. This was when Kent Brantly and Nancy Writebol returned to the US and Ebola appeared in Nigeria. This was when concerns of risk—spread, contagion, and the wider effects—started to infuse public debates. As the previous chapter noted, it was at this point when the distant tragedy of the outbreak became a *security* concern.

Beyond the timing, the securitizing discourses and their interaction also informed the *nature* of the response, both domestically and internationally. Again, we move here beyond the detail outlined in the previous chapter (how practices shifted and aligned with the rhetoric around it, as part of the securitizing discourses) to consider the response as a whole. Two attributes are notable here. First, although initial descriptions of the outbreak and response highlighted the suffering of West Africans and the need to save them, the response ultimately took a form closer to that of containment. As the four previous findings demonstrate, this was a process of securitization defined by risk logics, debates over authority and audience, and the threat of the inferior West African Other. Together, they constructed the outbreak predominantly (but not exclusively) as one of a possible foreign (African) threat to the US, with a terrified audience demanding sovereign action and certainty that the Obama administration and its experts were not providing. *This* was the emergency being responded to.

Accordingly, practices slowly adhered to notions of containment and were even explicitly labeled as such by the White House (2015). The emphasis in West Africa was on building Ebola treatment units and field laboratories and on providing full personal protective equipment and training. All of these were necessary but *temporary* and aimed less at immediately eliminating the outbreak (or addressing the reasons for the outbreak) than containing it. Moreover, the Obama administration staunchly refused to allow medical personnel within the military treat Ebola patients or transport them, which was justified, praised, and criticized as an effort to protect American lives first (Nevin and Anderson 2016, 55–56; Kamradt-Scott et al. 2015, 15). In the US, meanwhile, fifty-one specialized Ebola treatment centers were built, and enhanced airport screenings were implemented, with significant cost and little result (only one entrant out of approximately thirty-eight thousand was determined to have Ebola). Notably, the latter was described by the CDC itself as a change due to "public concern" and "in response to assertions that self-monitoring was insufficient" (Cohen et al.

2016, 60). Moreover, the CDC—and the Obama administration—refrained from explicitly criticizing actions by state authorities that went beyond CDC guidelines (such as enforced quarantine), even describing these as a "minimum standard" that could be exceeded (Cohen et al. 2016, 60).

It remains important not to be categorical about this. There is a tendency within some securitization work to claim that securitization inherently leads to such practices (Aradau 2004), but the existence of the HWA discourse and the overlap between this and the PGC discourse at points during the process of securitization demonstrates that security does not automatically lead to containment. The refusal to ban travelers from West Africa, the public and political challenges to health worker quarantine, and the insistence on continued testing and access to pharmaceuticals for West Africans all speak to the existence of nuance and multiplicity within the response. Yet these still became bound by a regime of truth that narrowed the conditions of possibility, with no long-term health system capacity building occurring and West African and health worker bodies still subjected to extra surveillance and confinement. As João Nunes (2016, 550) has argued, this was ultimately a "reduction" of the Ebola outbreak to a "discrete crisis event" and a Western security threat, one to be contained and solved.

Related to this is the second aspect of the response as a whole: its neglect of Ebola. This may seem contradictory, considering the media attention on the outbreak, but neglect is a wider phenomenon than just the absence of attention. It also means the absence of *care*. As Nunes (2016, 550) describes it, neglect refers to "the invisibility of the groups most affected by the disease, as well as of the social and economic conditions that made the outbreak possible." The understanding of the outbreak through the representations of Africa as the Dark Continent, the return to the solipsistic understanding of health security, and the construction of security via risk all served to obscure the West Africans suffering from the virus and erase any serious consideration of the wider conditions (beyond reiterating West African Fragility). As both Nunes (2016, 550) and Mark Honigsbaum (2017, 285) point out, this was not limited to public rhetoric but infused the response itself. Again, there was a lack of long-term health system capacity building. Moreover, depictions of West Africans as ignorant, believing in superstition, and relying excessively on unsafe traditions missed that community resistance was grounded in a history of colonial medical encounters, more recent relationships (including civil war) with their governments, and contemporary experiences with fragmented and expensive health systems (Benton and Dionne 2015; Fairhead 2015; Cohn and Kutalek 2016). The combination of these factors with the treatment of the outbreak as a Western security concern meant that community engagement was not prioritized and did not occur until later in the response (Honigbaum 2017, 286). By this point, however, locals were avoiding health facilities and violent clashes between locals and foreign health workers had already occurred.

To conclude, it is worth again reiterating the possibilities within this process of securitization and the response it formed. At various points, different responses became viable. Kent Brantly and Nancy Writebol might have been denied their return to the US due to fears of contagion. Experimental treatments might have been kept solely to Americans, while legal requirements for pharmaceutical research and development might have been loosened entirely. The military might not have been deployed or it might have been deployed with an expanded mandate, including patient care and long-term capacity building. A travel ban might have been enacted. Airport screening might have remained with its focus on self-monitoring and questionnaires. Kaci Hickox might have been forced to remain in her initial quarantine. There are many spaces in which different practices might have been enacted. Examining the interplay between the multiple securitizing discourses—and the key sites of contestation between them—provides us understanding as to why these choices were made, but it is vital to remember that these choices were never *determined*. Security actors operate within the conditions of possibility crafted by discourse, but they retain agency to act within them. In our critiques of health emergency response, we must remember this. We must critically consider both those involved in direct response (politicians, experts), those involved in constructing these regimes of truth that constrain and enable action (such as the media), and the agency of both as they interact.

Securitization beyond Ebola

It is here that the insights from the US response to Ebola begin to stretch further than just this case study. The sites of commonality and contestation discussed above do speak immediately to the Ebola case and then to the wider field of global health, but they also provide crucial insight into securitization itself: how it operates, what leads to success, and what it offers to our understanding of non-traditional security. In this section, I translate the case study findings into insights—or perhaps provocations—for the theory itself. This involves a return to the discussion in the first chapter, which examined the base Copenhagen School theory, delved into the second-generation literature that expanded, critiqued, and revised it, and used this to outline a discursive set up for analysis with a reconceptualization of security in terms of the "thick signifier" and the expanded logic of exceptionalism. There, I considered what the wider securitization literature gave to my study of pluralism and process in securitization. Here, I consider the major findings my study of pluralism and process gives back to this literature.

Contextual Discourses as Key to Meaning Production

Context is widely understood as important to securitization—The Copenhagen School refers to context as "facilitating conditions" (Buzan et al. 1998, 32). Beyond this, however, context's precise role in securitization remains nebulous. Others have stepped in to fill this gap. Thierry Balzacq (2005, 182), for instance, proposes that context's role is decisive for "resonance": it is only through connecting a claim to security with a prospective threat's "external reality" that said move can be accepted as truth. Felix Ciută (2009) takes this a step further in arguing that context is integral to the very construction of security's meaning and practice. Linking to Nils Bubandt's (2005) work on "vernacular security," Ciută (2009) highlights the need to consider "local political histories" of security and their role in securitizing moves. Ultimately, the construction of security is deeply entwined with—and perhaps even reliant on—the preexisting understandings and meanings actors have. This goes beyond mere facilitation and sees context as having a key role in meaning production itself.

The Ebola analysis reaffirms this. Contextual narratives of identity, disease, and security were crucial components of each securitizing discourse. The Self/Other relationship and the contestation over it were entwined with divergent understandings of the US as the Indispensable Nation, disease as a threat or a humanitarian concern, and Africa as the Dark Continent, all of which have long histories in American foreign policy and the American public understanding of itself and the African Other. Another key contextual narrative that provided meaning is what Priscilla Wald (2008, 2, 268) has termed the *outbreak narrative*, "an evolving story of disease emergence" that has "scientific, journalistic, and fictional incarnations" and follows a "formulaic plot" of an emerging infection, its spread across an interconnected world, its epidemiological tracing, and (hopefully) it's eventual containment through "the triumph of science and epidemiology". In a general sense, it is a narrative about the perils and possibilities of human interdependence and what relation the microbial has to it. Ebola and the US response fit easily into this basic narrative structure; indeed, it had already been positioned within it by Reston's *The Hot Zone* and the 1994 film *Outbreak*, both of which were drawn on by US political and media actors. We can also highlight the role of other contextual narratives: the immigration emphasis and the rise of Mexico as a possible source for contagion, the continued aversion to federal government control over private and state-level action, the "opportunistic politician" representation particularly prominent in the Fearbola counterdiscourse, and the understanding of the US military as both a uniquely humanitarian actor and a referent object in itself (encapsulated in the worry over "boots on the ground"). These contextual narratives existed prior to the Ebola outbreak, and they persist now in relation to other issues. Here, however, they intertwined with the claims to Ebola as a security issue, giving it a foundation already known and taken for granted and thus making it understandable.

Yet the Ebola analysis also speaks to the benefit of moving beyond the insistence of some second-generation scholars to view context as "external reality" or a single "political history" that gives securitization meaning. Objectivizing context in this way would miss the multiplicity and instability that was apparent in claims to context. The indispensability of the US, for instance, was understood variously: in one form, it spoke to American superiority and its inherent value to be protected, yet in another it demanded an obligation to the inferior Other. The outbreak narrative, speaking to the wider threat of "emerging infections," was similarly varied, with AUT proponents employing it to ground their claims of Ebola's risk to "us," while PGC advocates drew on its previous iterations (SARS, HIV/AIDS, etc.) to "remind" their audiences of the international turbulence that follows disease. Such an approach to context even highlights further agency in securitization, with critics from the Fearbola perspective using the outbreak narrative self-reflexively, pointing to its recurrences in the media and its role in curating the story of Ebola to fit this preexisting plot, as they also did the Dark Continent discourse (Kidjo 2014; Seay and Dionne 2014). And it was in this multiplicity that contestation between the discourses was perhaps the most rife, as they spoke to differing truths about the US, the world, and the threat of disease. In this vein, the securitization of Ebola was not simply a debate over the outbreak and its response but one of who/what the US is, what it values, and what its relationship to the world looks like.

Contextual discourses are therefore key to meaning production but are not simple explanations for it. They are not causes; indeed, even labeling them "facilitating conditions" ascribes to them a stability that context does not have. They are offered as taken-for-granted truths, foundational narratives of American public discourse, and even core values of the American people, but their precise meaning depends on how they are articulated. There is thus an important interplay between contextual and securitizing discourses, with the former providing meaning to the latter but also being (re)produced in the process. They are thus neither reducible to these articulations nor completely extractable. Analyzing securitizing discourses requires illuminating and examining this process of reiteration. Doing so enables an exploration of how context "works" in securitization without closing the process to the kinds of change and contestation that this analysis has highlighted.

Recognizing the Potential of Security's Meaning and Logic

This case study also offers some important insight into discussions around the concept at the heart of securitization theory: security. The first chapter noted the Copenhagen School's approach to security as historically sedimented in meaning and exceptionalist in its logic and practice. As that chapter outlined, a large number of security scholars from a variety of perspectives—the Paris School, risk, Foucauldian governmentality, and simply those examining security in practice—have revealed this to be an arbitrary limitation of security to an a priori definition. Yet there remains insight in the arguments of sedimentation and exceptionalism. As that chapter argued, we must try to find a way to move beyond the limitations while keeping these valuable ideas. The Ebola analysis reiterates this but provides two specific and important insights to the wider literature on security in securitization theory.

First, it reiterates that security's "thickness" remains just that: thick. Constructing and stabilizing a competing meaning to the concept—affirming the signifying capacity of security, in other words—remains a difficult endeavor. The sharpest divergence from this thick meaning of security was that of the HWA discourse, which linked the signifier of security to the long-term protection of distant individuals. Yet the HWA discourse was also the least prominent of the securitizing discourses. This is more than a correlation; the HWA discourse's challenge to the traditional friend/enemy relationship and the containment practices associated with externalized threat were the central points of contestation it faced. Take, for instance, Obama's speeches to the CDC and UN, where he asserted that the US could (and should) "save countless lives" in West Africa. While he also presented the threat in terms of the indirect potential catastrophe that could result, his formulation of the danger in terms that did not align with the immediate defense of the state drew ire, namely from those who compared it to the "most dangerous" issues, like ISIS (Eric Bolling, in The Five 2014a). Others simply reiterated these claims in ways that returned the signifier of security to its historically sedimented meaning, including even Obama (2015) himself.

Yet it remains important not to overstate this problem or claim that security inevitably falls back into exclusion, violence, and militarization. Despite being unable to overcome the "thickness" of security, the HWA discourse occupied a crucial role in contesting and expanding the opposing discourses. The West African referent was never entirely absent from the discussion; though diminished and neglected, it could not be completely dismissed and even became central at key points, notably the debates over experimental treatments and the threat of returning health workers. It is also striking that, as the politics of the AUT and PGC discourses became apparent following the midterms, the HWA discourse resurged as the apolitical, moral, and true representation of the outbreak's danger. The merging of the HWA discourse with the Fearbola counterdiscourse, and the success of this construction, is worth highlighting here. Perhaps its lesson is that alternative discourses of security operate best when they explicitly engage their position as alternatives to the thick understanding of security, highlighting the capacity to understand security differently.

The second, and perhaps more vital, insight regards security's logic: exceptionalism. Within this analysis, each securitizing discourse was identified in making a claim to Ebola's exceptional nature: the extremity of its threat, the necessity of immediate, urgent, and extraordinary action, and the role of a sovereign figure in deciding and centralizing power. Each suggested that Ebola necessitated an alteration to the current state of things or a change in its meaning and practice. Yet each understood this exceptional nature and the precise form of the exception it demanded differently. Crucially, none of these exceptions aligned neatly with the one that the Copenhagen School's formulation of securitization theory is grounded on: that of Carl Schmitt. The Ebola case thus reaffirms not only exceptionalism's potential for differing and multiple formulations but also the limitations in rigidly adhering to Schmittian exceptionalism as the center of security's logic.

Specifically, as noted earlier in the chapter, the Ebola case reiterates the need to recognize risk as a logic of exceptionalism. As that earlier section demonstrated, risk was central to the proposed definitions of security and to the claims of Ebola's exceptional nature and the exceptional response it ostensibly demanded. The AUT discourse, for instance, was premised on the idea that the possibility of an Ebola outbreak in the US was untenable and therefore required extraordinary action, including that which disrupted the political, legal, and civil norm: "there is a broad understanding at the Food and Drug Administration that this is no ordinary time, correct?" (Michael Burgess, in CFA 2014a, 74). The PGC discourse similarly focused on the future danger of Ebola but also highlighted the temporal (not imminent) and spatial (not direct) distance, which required alterations to (global and domestic) normality in the forms of preparedness and health systems rather than just short-term transgressions (though it suggested forms of this as well). Considering exceptionalism as a spectrum of political possibility as suggested in the first chapter, where exceptionalism is understood in terms of questions of intensity (the real possibility of violent death), transgression (the questioning of political limits), and authority (the decision and sovereign power), these claims to risk fit the mold. It was the risk of Ebola, its potential future harm, and the need to alter the norm that necessitated urgent and meaning-altering—exceptional—action.

The contentiousness of such an argument cannot be understated. As mentioned earlier, positioning risk within securitization has been disputed directly by Wæver. The core reason is exceptionalism. Risk is widely understood as the antithesis to Schmittian exceptionalism: the "mundane" to the "extraordinary," the "dispersed" to the "centralised," and the "everyday" to the "emergency" (Aradau et al. 2008; Corry 2012). As Huysmans (2011) has aptly highlighted, risk is ultimately a challenge to the politics enacted through claims to security and, accordingly, how we analyze and critique it. Securitization emphasizes the Schmittian exception in order to focus on moments of decisional gravity, where the norm is "ruptured" and "new possibilities of what is right and wrong" come into being (Huysmans 2011, 374–375). Yet the practices of risk—the dispersed, everyday, and governmentalizing "little security nothings"—efface the very idea of decisional gravity. Rather than dramatically "disrupting" a given order, they gradually and dispersedly "create" one (Huysmans 2011, 377–378). There is therefore the risk that we miss the significance of this logic while also blunting the incisive instrument aimed to capture the other. The differences between these logics are indeed crucial, as the Ebola case demonstrates. Contestation raged over them: whether the goal was to eliminate or manage danger, what kind of sovereign was necessary, and what basis of knowledge should be acted on. Yet, as the Ebola case also demonstrates, the notion that some of these were not claims to exceptionalism would be just as misguided as suggesting they were all the same kind. There is thus a need to consider how risk can operate as a form of exceptionalism without simply blurring it into the Schmittian analysis that securitization focuses on and thus losing its distinctive contribution.

I contend that the best way to do this is to emphasize risk as the opposing end of the exceptionalist spectrum.[1] Risk, like security, remains focused on the politics of emergency unleashed by the construction of danger. It maintains that the fear of the enemy operates as the constitutive principle of politics (Aradau and van Munster 2009, 689), highlighting the role of future harm (whether imminent or possible) in legitimizing exceptional behavior and state mobilization. And its scholars are just as concerned with how technologies of risk entrench governmental power over populations as the securitization literature is with speech acts (Lund Petersen 2011, 701–702; see also Bigo 2002; Aradau and van Munster 2007; Elbe 2008; Salter 2008a). The difference, however, is that the Schmittian exception locates this exception as a separate space, one invoked by the sovereign decision, while risk folds the exception back into normality rather than separating the two. As Aradau et al. (2008, 152) summarize it, risk "infuses exceptionalism within the governmentality of everydayness." This is most evident in risk's emphasis on bureaucratic and technological management, which is ultimately the routinization of emergency practices, the dispersal of the decision among multiple actors, and the alteration of the norm to accommodate them. Exceptionalism, however, is not simply risk or security; it is a spectrum of politics between the Schmittian extreme and the most mundane forms of risk management.

This brings us to perhaps the most novel insight this empirical analysis revealed: exceptionalism's potential for multiple forms can be observed within one single claim to exceptionalism. It was in the positions between those traditionally defined as risk and security that the securitizing discourse of Ebola staked themselves. Each discourse merged the risk and security logics into more complex, nuanced, and even occasionally contradictory claims. The AUT discourse, with its emphasis on possibility derived from speculating from uncertainty, still insisted on a direct existential threat that required the centralizing of decisional power within a sovereign and the extreme rupture to the American democratic (and legal) norm. In this vein, the risk of Ebola demanded the invocation of a Schmittian exception. Meanwhile, the PGC and HWA discourses both focused on certainty, albeit to varying degrees. The PGC discourse was centered on a risk as well, and the exception it sought to produce was far more in line with the gradual order-altering associated with the risk logic. But it also implemented practices aligned closer to the Schmittian exception: the deployment of the US military and the breaking of pharmaceutical regulations, for instance. Indeed, early formulations of the PGC discourse were frequently linked to the clear imminent threat the HWA discourse focused on, looking to combine the risk of global insecurity to the threat for West Africa in order to heighten the exceptional circumstance of the outbreak. The HWA discourse, however, did insist on an imminent direct threat (to West Africa) and an emergency response (in West Africa) but also highlighted that the issue was the lack of appropriate normality rather than the excess of it. Emergency responses were therefore needed but not enough; a long-term approach of managing health issues was required. Accordingly, each of the securitizing discourses constructed an exception that saw the mundane and the speculative as entwined with the exceptional and the imminent. Understanding these discourses requires a consideration of this entwining, not its arbitrary separation.

More crucially, however, it was in the entwining of these logics that contestation raged. The AUT discourse rejected the PGC and HWA discourses' assertion that the risk of hypothetical travelers could simply be managed.

The PGC and HWA discourses challenged the notion that an extreme disruption to civil liberties (such as mandatory quarantining or closing borders) was permissible on the basis of a hypothetical threat. Yet the PGC and HWA discourses also contested each other on what kind of exception was required, where it should be located (and where it should not), and to what degree. This can be observed, for instance, in the worries that the US's frantic building of centers was out of touch with what West Africans really needed (Bernstein 2014) and the concerns that the Obama administration would diminish its role once the global risk seemed to have been managed (Ban 2014; Gladstone 2014; Coons 2015). These were not cases of risk versus security, but they did touch on some of the tensions between them, namely the issues of management versus elimination, the breaking of norms versus their alteration, and the demand for a gravitational decision versus the efficacy and validity of "little security nothings." Ultimately, Huysmans and Corry are right to note that there are key political differences between the claims associated with the Schmittian exception and those of risk that should not be ignored. Yet removing this entirely from exceptionalism would be to deny the very basis they do share and, most crucially, where these differences engage, contest, and align with one another.

Securitization as Process

Before concluding this chapter, it is worth reiterating one of the core insights of this book as a whole: securitization must be understood and analyzed as a political process. It is not a single moment of speech by a predefined securitizing actor. It is not a single acceptance by a clear audience. It is not the enactment of a single emergency measure. The US response to Ebola demonstrates it as a reiterative and productive process with multiple claims to security (variously defined) that intersect, contest, and change. It involves many actors, all with varying claims to institutional and social authority: political sovereign, expert, bureaucrat, Heroic Health Worker, journalist, and so on. It is shaped by its context, drawing on prominent domestic narratives of identity and security, yet it is also not determined by it, with each of these reproduced and altered in the process. It manifests in varying kinds of exceptionalism, from the mundane kinds of risk management to the extremes of war. These emergency measures reiterate these constructions, but they also feed back into this process, becoming new sites for debate. Securitization may indeed be the exception, or the "passage to the limit"

(Huysmans 1998b, 571), but it is always one grounded in the normal political realm in which it is enacted. It is a political process. And in analyzing it as such, this book provides two important insights about securitization.

First, we must pay attention to how multiplicity and contestation operate within domestic cases of securitization. The Copenhagen School framework's inability to account for different meanings and practices of security has been extensively explored (see Bubandt 2005; Trombetta 2008; Ciută 2009). Yet even with the numerous alternative approaches to securitization offered, relatively little of this work has considered how these multiple meanings might operate within the one domestic case. As this book's analysis demonstrates, this can be core to securitization. The securitizing discourses within the US securitization of Ebola formed in relation to one another. The AUT discourse's representations of threat, referent, audience, and authority shifted as it was contested by HWA proponents in the early stages of August, while the PGC discourse was first uttered in ways that drew on the exception as outlined by the HWA discourse but also altered it. They interacted at the level of key representations, competing and overlapping in their claims to threat, referent, audience, authority, context, and security's meaning and practice. They shifted as a response, with particular representations (West Africans as referent) becoming less viable and others (the American people as referent) demanding adherence or response. In accordance, the response itself shifted, with the military deployed, travelers screened, quarantines enacted and revoked, and money spent. Indeed, we must remember that this emphasis on securitization as a process goes beyond just academic interest in understanding securitization. These domestic competitions over meaning—what a threat is, who is threatened, what we value, who we are, who should act, and how—inform global responses, including to some of our most pressing threats.

Secondly, actors have the capacity to be self-reflexive and critical about securitization within the process of securitizing. As Colin McInnes and Simon Rushton (2013, 127–131) have argued in relation to HIV/AIDS, actors can partially accept securitization or accept it at one point and reject it at another. We might add to this the capacity for actors to alter their precise positions on securitization as they move between different securitizing discourses or change their practices. News anchors, media commentators, and reporters in particular jumped between concern for West Africa, worrying about the risk to the US, lamenting the impacts on the economy and

regional stability, and mocking such concerns. By focusing on securitizing discourses rather than single speech acts, these shifts can be read as
actors navigating the discursive terrain and the conditions of possibility.
We can also consider within this approach the (likely) possibility that some
actors may have purposefully engaged securitizing narratives for electoral
reasons, particularly in their campaigns for the midterms. The sudden drop
in attention to Ebola after the elections suggests this. What is perhaps most
striking, however, is the apparent confirmation this analysis provides to
Michael C. Williams's (2011) idea of the "securitization of securitization."
Drawing from Judith Shklar's (1998) "liberalism of fear," Williams (2011,
454) argues that liberal societies are aware of the deleterious effects of fear
on liberal politics: the excesses and "institutionalized cruelty" that security
can foment. They thus fear the politics of fear and can use this fear to act as
a "bulwark against such processes," even by securitizing securitization itself
(Williams 2011, 456). The Ebola case, particularly the Fearbola counterdiscourse, offers some empirical validation for this claim. Ultimately, what
we can observe from this is the importance of considering agency within
securitization and agency beyond just the sovereign.

Conclusion

This chapter sought to explicitly combine the empirical analysis of the past
two chapters with the theoretical discussion in the first. Two goals were
paramount here. First, we needed to draw together the previous two chapters to consider just what they revealed about the US response to Ebola.
Four key findings were outlined in the first section of this chapter. First,
the Self/Other construction was a key commonality between the discourses
and, as such, was also a key site for contestation. Second, the construction of an accepting audience and its connected constructions of authority (political, expert, and moral) were central to both constructing security
and the contestation around it. Third, the constructions of security within
the securitizing discourses were deeply informed by logics of risk in their
meaning and practice, and the precise linkages between risk and security
were varied and contested. And finally, this contested domestic process of
securitization resulted in a US response to Ebola that was late, focused on
containment, and ultimately reinscribed the neglect of Ebola and those
who suffer its effects the most.

The second goal was to consider what this offers back to securitization studies and the enormous body of critical scholarship within it. Here, I focused on the three major contributions this book provides to some of the key debates within the wider securitization literature. First, I reiterated the nuanced role of contextual discourses in meaning production. They are central to securitization, drawn on as taken-for-granted truths about one's identity, those of Others, what we value, and how we should act. Yet they are—like all discourses—unstable and require reiteration. They can shift and change in this reiteration, given meaning by securitization just as they give meaning to it. Second, the meaning and logic of security must be recognized for their sedimentation, exceptionalism, *and* their capacity to differ. Security's meaning remains thick: historically sedimented and difficult to alter. Yet alterations do exist and have impact in processes of securitization, as the HWA discourse demonstrates. Similarly, while the Copenhagen School's emphasis on Schmitt remains valid, the concept of exceptionalism must be expanded to cover a spectrum of political possibility, specifically the role of risk. Finally, securitization must be understood as a process. Domestic contests over identity and threat, containing multiple perspectives and positions, shape global responses. Actors, meanwhile, retain agency and a capacity for self-reflexivity. As a theoretical approach that seeks to understand the construction of security, securitization theory must capture this plurality.

6 Conclusion: Global Health beyond Ebola

The 2014–2015 West African outbreak of Ebola was, as President Obama (2014d) outlined on September 2014, "more than a health crisis." For Obama, this spoke to his understanding—an understanding eventually shared by most other US policymakers, members of the media, and the general public—that the outbreak was a threat to *security*. It demanded an urgent reconsideration of how we understood the disease and the legal, ethical, and institutional boundaries in which we could and should act. This was, as many international relations scholars analyzing this case have suggested, a clear case of securitization, where an issue is constructed as a security threat through the representation of it as such.

Yet Obama's labeling of the outbreak as "more than a health crisis" is pertinent for more than its immediate meaning. For the US, the Ebola outbreak was not only more than a health crisis in the sense of it also being a security crisis but also in the simple fact that it was more than just a crisis about a disease outbreak. It was also a crisis about American identity and (West) African identity. It was a crisis about power and authority, about Obama's presidency and the Democrat/Republican divide. It was about the dangers of a globalized world and the role of the United States and its military within it. Accordingly, the US response to Ebola was entwined with these domestic and global issues and, as a result, contested. A variety of political and media actors made multiple, competing claims to security, drawing on long-running contextual narratives, different forms of authority, domestic debates about immigration and practice, and logics of risk and security to produce different understandings of the outbreak and its threat. While it remains apt to say that Ebola was securitized within the US, it was never neatly securitized. There was no single securitizing speech act, moment of audience acceptance, and clear emergency measures. Instead, there was a complex, messy, and *deeply political* debate about what kind of threat Ebola might pose, who it might threaten, in what way, who knew this threat, who should act, and what they should do.

This book has explored this plurality and contestation as a discursive process of securitization, as outlined in the first chapter ("Setting up Securitization"). It mapped the different securitizing discourses and counter-discourse evident in the US political and media landscape (in "The Basic Securitizing Discourses") and traced the interaction between them (in "Securitizing Ebola") over the key months of the US response to the outbreak: July 2014 to February 2015. In doing so, it demonstrated that the America Under Threat (AUT) discourse—an understanding of the outbreak as a threat to the US homeland—ultimately dominated this debate, particularly when it counted in September to November 2014. As argued in the last chapter ("Securitizing beyond Ebola"), the AUT discourse's dominance can be understood through its reproduction of a powerful contextual discourse regarding the Self/Other relationship, namely the construction of the (West) African Other as a source of threat (or enemy), its construction of a fearful audience, its challenges to the political, moral, and expert authorities other discourses relied on, and its conceptualization of security through the Schmittian extreme combined with the uncertainty and speculation of risk. This resulted in a response to Ebola that was late, focused primarily on containment, and ultimately re-entrenched the neglect of Ebola and West Africa. As this chapter then argued, this speaks to key insights for securitization theory, namely the nuanced centrality of contextual discourses in informing not only threat but also who gets to be the referent object, who and what the audience is and values, what authority looks like, and what kind of emergency measures can be implemented as well as the need to consider risk as a logic of exceptionalism.

Yet it is vital to remember that while the AUT discourse dominated this process of securitization, it did not *define* it. We can only understand what happened, how, and why through considering the interplay between the discourses. The AUT discourse did not always guide the response. The Potential Global Catastrophe discourse remained an important counterposition, even as the Obama administration shifted closer to the AUT discourse. Travel bans and health worker quarantines continued to be contentious. The Helpless West Africa discourse kept West Africans in the story. Their suffering could never be completely dismissed. The Fearbola counterdiscourse, moreover, effectively undermined the AUT discourse in November. This is perhaps the basic empirical argument of this book: the US securitization of Ebola must be understood as a process of contestation between these three securitizing discourses and the counterdiscourse.

At least, that is the basic empirical argument regarding the US securitization of Ebola. So far, this book has focused almost exclusively on this case, while also discussing the implications for securitization theory. In this concluding chapter, however, I will take this analysis up a level: to the securitization of disease and global health security in general. What does this detailed, focused examination of the US response to Ebola tell us about global health security, namely some of the biggest problems we face in outbreak and pandemic response? What does the securitization of Ebola demonstrate about the securitization of disease? What does it tell us about how we view disease more generally? What insights might we take, for instance, to address the elephant in the room: the COVID-19 pandemic? This final chapter will consider these questions, drawing from the book's analysis of the US response to Ebola to consider the larger global health story it sits within.

Global Health Security as Glimpsed through Ebola

The Promise and Problems of Medical Expertise

We start specific, engaging one of the most prominent issues in global health responses: the contested role of expertise. Despite their differences, disease outbreaks and pandemics sit alongside issues like climate change and nuclear weapons in one crucial way: they are scientifically complex, uncertain, and potentially dangerous problems. The average layperson struggles to understand the significance of a new pathogen, the spread of an old one, the rise in global temperatures, or the creation of a new weapon delivery system. We rely on experts—those trained in these areas—to communicate the problems and how to respond to them adequately. Expert knowledge has perhaps never been more crucial. Yet it has also perhaps never been more contested. Whether we call this the "crisis of expertise" (Eyal 2019), the "death of expertise" (Nichols 2017), or the rise of "post-truth politics," we are increasingly aware of how experts are questioned, mistrusted, debated, and outright dismissed. Within global health security, where medical experts are crucial to identifying and responding to threats, this problem is particularly acute. This book's analysis of the US response to Ebola offers two important insights into this crisis of expertise as it manifests in relation to global health emergencies.

First, it illuminates the question of who gets to be an expert within such debates. The experts drawn on were largely those of established medical or public health positions, such as the director of the CDC, the head of the NIAID, and university professors (with these titles often emphasized). Yet in-house medical correspondents were also represented as expert authorities, with Dr. Sanjay Gupta (CNN), Dr. Mark Siegel (Fox), and Dr. Nancy Snyderman (MSNBC/NBC) often called on to offer a decisive word on events and policies. In the last chapter, I outlined medical/expert authority as defined by two things: expertise and neutrality. We might also frame these as medical knowledge and institutional recognition. Knowledge from other experts, such as anthropologists, was rarely drawn on. Medical professionals in general—by virtue of having medical knowledge—were occasionally able to comment,[1] but most experts were those who were institutionally recognized (and thus seen as neutral). A particular gap here, however, is that of local health workers and public health experts. Most quoted experts, even in reporting from West Africa, were foreign health workers; only a few locals were asked to comment on the crisis befalling their communities.[2]

The question of who gets to be an expert is a vital one for two reasons. First, we have seen a proliferation of voices within this expert space, including those who lack the training or experience to speak on particular topics. We must ask ourselves why particular people are placed in this position of authority. Do they actually have expertise? Do they work within the relevant field? Are they recognized by their peers as experts? Secondly, it informs whose knowledge is worth knowing and acting on. As a number of scholars have since pointed out, this denial of local expertise and community knowledge also appeared in the response in West Africa (Caremel et al. 2016, 74–75; Honigsbaum 2017). Sophie Harman (2016) has similarly pointed to the "conspicuous invisibility" of women during the Ebola response, where their labor in the care economy was vital for the response but they were missing from its strategies, policy, and practice. Clare Wenham (2021, 3–4) has similarly argued that global health security "neglects women's reality," particularly that of poorer women of color. As she argues, this is solved not by simply adding more women to the table but by considering feminist perspectives and expertise.

The second insight derives from the first: how expertise is contested. This connects to the two sources for authority mentioned above: expertise (knowledge) and neutrality (institution). The Ebola case showed medical expertise contested through a claim that they were so focused on what was known, certain, and likely that they did not consider the unknown, uncertain, and unlikely. This may seem a catch-22 for experts, who are called on to communicate what is known and not known, judge the risk, and offer the best solutions. There is a crucial process of weighting that occurs here: the likelihood of a risk against the devastation it might cause. Yet as Claudia Aradau and Rens van Munster (2011) have argued, contemporary security concerns are increasingly dominated by the unlikely catastrophe. Here, the catastrophe's possible devastation is so great as to minimize the importance of its (un)likelihood. *Imagination* thus becomes a key security practice, where the most unlikely futures are drawn into the present as the basis for action. Speculation, of course, has always been part of risk calculation, but this shift toward uncertainty and imagination as the basis for this speculation take us beyond the usual management of risk (de Goede 2008, 156). When we consider this within health emergencies, particularly an outbreak where the culprit disease is both horrible and largely unknown by the audience, this problem of imagination can be particularly damning for experts. Indeed, in this case, the AUT discourse not only demonstrates this power of imagination in threat construction but also, crucially, illuminates how this emphasis on the "what if" can be used to destabilize the authority of those who seek to communicate the "what is."

This case also showed how institutional recognition can operate *against* expert authority. The CDC, for instance, was battered by suggestions that it was politically contaminated due to its position as a government agency. Frieden's position as a government official, working alongside Obama, was used to present his knowledge as tainted, as simply the whims of the Obama administration. Of course, expertise is always political. As Anna Leander and Ole Wæver (2018, 2–3) define it, expertise is not science or knowledge in and of itself. It is the *application* of this knowledge to a problem. There are inevitably choices and values at play in how a problem is understood and which solutions are deemed best. Moreover, experts must operate within structures, including alongside government, to be recognized and perform this "knowledge work" (Kennedy 2016, 110). What this case demonstrates is an inability to constructively engage the politics of expertise. Rather than consider how expertise may always be political and what this means for a response, we simply hold it up against an idealized apolitical form of expertise. As Sheila Jasanoff and Hilton R. Simmet (2017, 765) have aptly noted, this effectively means that scientific challenges are suggested to be political disputes and political debates can masquerade as scientific ones. AUT proponents used this effectively. Obama, Frieden, Fauci, and others did not deny a travel ban because of any *scientific certainty* that an outbreak was unlikely but because of their *politics*. Meanwhile, their demand for a travel ban was not a political challenge, aimed to undermine Obama's political authority prior to midterm elections, but one based on "common sense" science.

Both of these insights speak to current problems within global health. The authority of the world's most prominent expert body—the WHO—is tenuous. While a part of this lies in the organization's missteps, including in its response to Ebola (Kamradt-Scott 2018), it is also plagued by claims that it is a political entity, one "in bed" with big pharma or even a puppet for other states. These disputes typically revolve around its institutional position as an intergovernmental organization reliant on member-state funding. Rather than questioning what this means for the WHO's autonomy and capacity as an expert and technical body, this is used to dismiss its expertise altogether. Expert medical knowledge more generally has also been undermined. As Heidi J. Larson (2020) argues, a significant part of contemporary vaccine hesitancy lies in the mistrust populations feel toward the medical establishment and the way this feeds into their risk calculations, amplified as rumors. Ultimately, this book provides another angle to this story of the crisis of expertise as it appears in global health security. It illuminates how the politics of expertise manifest and operate within one of the main states responding to a global health emergency. It points to the choices made in who gets to speak, who is recognized to know, and who is heard. It outlines how actors can use these dismissal tactics for political advantage, as well as how other actors respond to and combat it. And perhaps most fundamentally, it points to how central these contests over expert authority are to a health security response.

Health Security as Discourse

These contests over expert authority relate to the second major contribution this book offers to our understanding of global health security: the value of examining health security through discourse. As the introduction outlined, multiple understandings of health security exist, with the national security approach tending to dominate over the policy and practice of global health security. In analyses of Ebola so far, some have taken these understandings as reasons for action. It was the prioritization of "collective vulnerability" over "individual health security" that lead to the international response's failure (Heymann 2016). It was the securitization of Ebola that led to the emphasis on pharmaceutical Magic Bullets (Roemer-Mahler and Elbe 2016), the militarization of the response (Benton 2016), and the continued neglect of Ebola and West Africa (Nunes 2016; Honigsbaum 2017). Others have noted different meanings at different levels, such as Christian Enemark's (2017a) examination of how the UN Security Council sought to secure circulation against states' more traditional national security approaches. These are all insightful contributions. Indeed, this book is built off such work, following their emphasis on the construction of meaning and the effects this has on shaping response.

Yet it also took a slightly different tack to this. In this book, I dove deep into the (re)construction of these understandings within a single state responder, perhaps one of the most prominent global health actors. I focused on how exactly health security was reproduced, including in different and competing forms. I analyzed how they interacted within this single context and how they changed in response to one another and the events that occurred. And I detailed not only how this formed the response of the US but also how it might have formed this response differently. This book, in other words, reveals the nuanced, complex, and contested power of discourse in shaping health security and emergency response.

Two important insights regarding health security derived from this focus. Firstly, it reiterates that global health security is not a uniform or static concept. As Clare Wenham (2019, 1095) argues, "the meanings of both 'health' and 'security' . . . have varied depending on the immediate pathogen posing a threat." As the book demonstrates, this variation can occur even in relation to the same pathogen. Multiple understandings of health security can be evident within one response. Moreover, these understandings can and do change, particularly as they contest and clash. These have clear impacts on a state's response to a disease outbreak. In addition, this book's analysis affirms a tendency toward discourses of risk and precaution that has been noted within global health security work (Elbe 2008; Weir and

Mykhalovskiy 2010; McInnes and Roemer-Mahler 2017; Kirk 2020), yet it also stresses how we must not replace our focus on security or the Schmittian exception with one on risk. In essence, this book demonstrates the value in examining just how health security is constructed in each instance. We must trace how health events emerge and are shaped through discourse, how representations of security are linked, how this manifests in practice, and how much contestation and change occurs through this process.

Securitization theory remains an insightful conceptual tool for this. The Copenhagen School's emphasis on the construction of security—specifically through the representations of threat, referent object, audience, security actor, and emergency measures—provides a useful analytical framework to analyze health security discourses. Second-generation securitization work also draws our attention to questions of authority, audience, and context. Together, they provide a parsimonious and effective framework. Indeed, this is core to why the framework remains so popular within the global health security literature, even when many have identified its limitations (Hameiri and Jones 2015). Moreover, the original theory provides a compelling theoretical argument, namely in its understanding of security through exceptionalism. It encourages scholars to delve into the political *consequences* of attaching security to a disease, particularly the way it establishes a "political modality" that allows the breaking of rules, laws, and norms and the expansion of government power over the lives, bodies, and livelihoods of populations (Nunes 2016c, 64; Elbe 2005, 2009). In essence, employing securitization theory encourages us to examine not only how health security discourses are constructed but the impacts they have.

Secondly, this book revealed just how *domestic* global health emergency responses are. While we might collectively proclaim an understanding of global health security that seems far removed from the petty partisanship and national interests of states, this book demonstrates how health security as it is practiced is shaped by contests around identity, values, power, and authority. The US response to Ebola was never just about Ebola or even global health. It was about Obama's presidency. It was about who the American people are and what they value. It was about the contemporary role of the US military. It was about immigration. It was about (West) Africa and its relationship to the US. It was about the level of trust the people had in the CDC and the NIH. It was about our fears of disease in general, and our concerns regarding globalization. Again, this links to the wider global health security literature, namely those who have identified the role of context and audience in the securitization of disease (Curley and Herington 2011; McInnes and Rushton 2011; Kamradt-Scott and McInnes 2012). Yet this book provides a crucial addition to this work: it reveals that context and audience are not single entities that act as explanations for a securitization process but sites of contest wherein the precise form of securitization is shaped and altered. To properly grasp why and how a disease outbreak is responded to in the way it is, we must therefore look beyond the disease to the society that is securitizing it.

As outlined in the introduction of this concluding chapter, the US response to Ebola was more than a health crisis. This is also an apt description of disease securitization and global health security as a whole. They are always about more than just the immediate health crisis. They are about power, knowledge, identity, authority, risk, history, and other domestic considerations. They are about how the rest of the world is understood and valued. And this results in multiple, competing understandings. It results in an approach to health security that does not always neatly follow the traditional meaning of national security nor the Schmittian logic of exception. In this vein, this book attests to the importance of considering securitization and discourse in our analysis of global health emergencies. The validity of securitization theory may remain contested, but the value of considering just how a disease outbreak becomes a security threat—and all of the messy, contested, and deeply political representations that are involved in this process—is enormous.

The Securitization of Disease: Race, Fear, Exception

Finally, this book furthers a long discussion on just how we live with dangerous diseases. It reiterates the tendency toward securitizing disease outbreaks and highlights what happens in these varying formulations of the nexus of disease and security. As others have aptly argued, disease outbreaks are frequently racialized, assumed as a confirmation of cultural or racial inferiority (Kraut 1995; Wald 2008, 8). The image of Africa as a dirty, diseased place lies at the heart of the Dark Continent discourse, a contextual frame that infused each of the securitizing discourses and underwrote the AUT discourse (and its dominance) in particular. We can even see this within discourses that sought to protect West Africans, with forms of the Helpless West Africa discourse falling into a representation of West Africans as passive, helpless sufferers. Yet it was not just Africa that received this treatment. We can observe this wider racialization within the easy linkage to immigration and the US-Mexico border in particular. Worries about Ebola patients getting to a neighboring country and "walk[ing] right in" or the potential hordes of infected patients should Ebola cause an outbreak there did not seem to extend to Canada, after all (Fox News 2014).

More generally, this book provides a glimpse into the unique nature of disease as a security threat. Some in the field of global health security have highlighted the significance of health security in terms of its push toward securing microbial life and biopolitics (Elbe 2005; 2014; Youde 2010). While this book does not go down the path of the "pharmaceuticalization" of security (see Elbe 2014, 2018), it does offer insight into how disease provokes an inward shift of security's focus. Ebola's threat was frequently described in personalized terms (either to the US audience or with West African individuals attached), with its symptoms depicted in graphic detail in order to invoke a visceral response from the audience. Its microbial nature was emphasized: it was invisible, hidden, and carried via the bodies of Others and infiltrated one's most intimate space—the body—without notice. Ebola was thus not simply recognized as threatening but was dreaded as violent, unstoppable, and unknowable. This uncertainty and dread of microbial life (and death) formed a potent mixture. It was linked to the demand for a greater amount of surveillance and control over individuals to protect the population overall, with the key visible relationship being between the microbe and the population, with the individual bodies in the middle (Kaci Hickox, Craig Spencer, the many travelers and health workers subjected to quarantines and enhanced screenings) lost or actively dismissed.

As Phillip Alcabes (2009, 10) writes, "our understanding of disease has evolved with the state of knowledge about how we are affected by nature, and it has borne a changing burden of anxieties about bodies, souls, and the way we live in the world we have made." Disease has been (and continues to be) used to signify divine punishment, retribution from the natural world, and moral contamination. The merging of this with security thus offers a confluence of fears—nature, bodies, souls, and the relationship we hold to them—mixed with the politics of exception, a politically volatile concoction. While this book demonstrates that nothing is completely determined from the outset on how this evolves, it also shows that the potential for combustion remains rife. Perhaps the starkest demonstration of this, and thus the perfect note to end on, is COVID-19.

The Elephant in the Room

This is, of course, not a book about COVID-19. Indeed, its purpose was to finally offer the Ebola response the in-depth examination it deserves. In doing so, however, it inevitably offers insights that can be drawn into our understanding of COVID-19, the responses to it, and the devastation the pandemic has caused. In fact, it could be said that any book about global health security after 2020 will be, in some way, a book about COVID-19, whether outlining the lessons we should have learned before the pandemic or the lessons we had learned that aided us when SARS-CoV-2 started spreading from Wuhan, China. Rather than ignore this elephant in the room, it is worth considering just what this analysis provides in understanding the response to COVID-19 as well as what it does not.

Firstly, while state-level responses to COVID-19 differed, one common strategy of many governments (particularly in the West) was to represent the pandemic as a security threat. Within the US, President Donald Trump referred to himself as a "wartime president" and repeatedly claimed the US response was akin to a "war" against COVID-19, which he also frequently labeled the "Chinese virus," rendering it a foreign invader (Bump 2020; Kirk 2022). We could thus consider the response one of securitization and, like the Ebola case, explore just what it means for responses to use the label of security. Some within the global health security literature have done just this, considering how the logic of security has necessitated practices such as bordering (Ferhani and Rushton 2020; Liu and Bennett 2020), the denial of civil liberties and human rights (Gozdecka 2021), and the expansion of policing (Parker et al. 2020; Stott et al. 2020), surveillance (van Kolfschooten and de Ruijter 2020), and government power (Molnár et al. 2020; Vankovska 2020; Hassan 2022). Others have used securitization theory to inquire as to the precise nature of these responses, examining whether this was an elite-driven securitization (Kirk and McDonald 2021), where exactly the threat was located (Murphy 2020; Nunes 2020), and the role of war metaphors as the mode of securitization (Caso 2020; Musu 2020).

From this book's analysis, we can draw parallels between the securitization of COVID-19 and that of Ebola, observing similarities and differences in how the health-security nexus was invoked. One similarity includes the fact that this securitization occurred in multiple, competing forms, and there was significant partisanship involved in which approach was taken by different actors. The precise nature of the threat was disputed, though rather than the referent object splitting between Americans, West Africans, and the nebulous notion of global and regional stability, COVID-19 saw Americans themselves split. Was the entire population threatened or was it "just" the elderly, the immunocompromised, and the disabled? The nature of the exception and its encroachment on the political norm was also disputed. Were stay-at-home orders and mask requirements justifiable or an unconscionable violation of personal liberties? Could we understand this as a "securitization of securitization," as I have argued elsewhere (Kirk 2022)? There is thus the same need to consider just how the disease was variously constructed as a security threat, including the role of context, constructions of the audience, processes of authorization, and questions concerning what kind of exception is most appropriate.

Other similarities are also apparent. The pandemic saw foreign bodies rendered threats, blocked from entering the US. Racialization recurred, with spikes in hate crimes committed against Asian Americans observed in the early stages of the pandemic and no less than the president referring to COVID-19 as "the Chinese virus" (van Rythoven 2020). The "strongman" politician representation—Chris Christie with Ebola, Donald Trump with COVID-19—was employed to construct authority and to challenge it, as critics claimed it a performance aimed at votes, not effective policy. The outbreak narrative was again apparent, with the Huanan Seafood Markets now the dirty and diseased place the disease originates from,[3] globalization the key to its spread, and vaccines and heroic scientists the solution. Yet there is a crucial twist in this story, one that speaks to a similar finding from the Ebola case: the two latter elements—vaccines and expertise—were not as widely accepted as the outbreak narrative might suggest. Indeed, this is perhaps one of the most important insights this book may offer to analysis of the US response to COVID-19: the powerful role of uncertainty and the failures to grasp the politics of expertise.

The COVID-19 pandemic, with a new and unknown disease at its core, is a perfect crisis of uncertainty. While SARS-CoV-2 was genetically mapped within a couple of weeks of it being identified as a novel coronavirus, its precise manifestations (and their severity), how exactly it spread, how best to stop it, and how to treat it remained unknowns (and debated) for many months. In the meantime, the disease spread extensively, and people sickened and died. A significant part of the early pandemic, therefore, is the lack of knowledge. This is distinctly unlike that of Ebola, a disease which was "discovered" in 1976, has had multiple virus types identified, and has been the cause of numerous outbreaks across various countries in Africa (though was not known to have had any in West Africa until 2014). Yet Ebola was also a crisis of uncertainty, though in the sense of manufactured uncertainty which highlighted the things that remained uncertain (vaccines and pharmaceuticals) and the unlikely possibilities (mutation). In both cases, speakers used this uncertainty both to rely on experts and to diminish them.

The Ebola case thus offers a detailed examination of how expertise is contested through speculation, uncertainty, and an inability to constructively contend with the politics of expertise. COVID-19 saw similar but slightly different manifestations of this. The real lack of information in the early stages meant that claims made during this time inevitably changed. One area of dispute surrounded the efficacy of mask wearing. Early in the pandemic, the level of asymptomatic cases was not known, so the benefits of mask wearing remained nebulous. Yet, even here, political considerations were at play. One concern of public health officials during this time was the lack of supplies and the prospect that people would purchase N95 masks desperately needed for health care workers. As supplies became more available and—more importantly—as information about how many people are asymptomatic with COVID-19 became known, this advice changed. Though this testifies to experts being attentive and responsive to how situations change, parts of the media and even the president himself represented this as a "mistake" and proof that they get things wrong (CNN 2020). This mistake was then used to dismiss current expertise: Fauci was wrong about masks early in the pandemic, so can *anything* he says be trusted?

Like the Ebola response, key expert authorities have been portrayed as politically contaminated, using science for their own political goals. In contrast, however, this meant they were represented as fearmongers, seeking to curtail American liberties (Mastrangelo 2020; Rutledge 2020). Other actors—including other medical professionals—have claimed expert authority for themselves by suggesting that they were offering the apolitical truth. Like Osterholm's mutation article in September 2014, they too have suggested that they were simply saying what "real" experts were saying secretly. For instance, Scott Atlas, a neuroradiologist whose commentary on Fox News led to President Trump recruiting him for the Coronavirus task force, proclaimed that data showed lockdowns and masks were actually useless (Abutaleb et al. 2020). We thus have, as Jasanoff and Simmet (2017, 760) summarize it, "my science versus yours" which masks the fact that this is ultimately a dispute over the more political aspects: whose lives are worth saving and what sacrifices we are willing to make for it.

Ultimately, between the Ebola and COVID-19 crises, we can observe a wider phenomenon within US politics regarding the role of science and knowledge more generally in decision and policy making. Some have labeled this "post-truth politics" or the "politicization of science," but it might perhaps be more accurate to consider this a problem of "scientization of politics" (Eyal 2019), where science is presented as the ultimate arbiter of policy value and the simple fact that political choices are made in the application of knowledge to a problem is presented as negative. This is not a new issue; debates over "junk science" can be traced back to the Reagan administration (Jasanoff and Simmet 2017, 756–759). Yet they take on a unique fervor when it comes to outbreaks and pandemics, perhaps because these cases invoke security and the exception it produces.

This speaks to one of the most interesting differences between the Ebola case and that of COVID-19 (especially in the US): Ebola saw much more agreement around the idea that the outbreak was threatening, while a significant problem within the US COVID-19 response was the refusal of particular key actors and large enough segments of the population to accept COVID-19's danger and the kinds of responses necessary to address it. We can even see elements of the "securitization of securitization" here: claims that COVID-19 policies such as stay-at-home orders and mask wearing are attempts by (Democrat) politicians and their expert puppets to expand their control over the populace, using the politics of fear (see Kirk 2022). Yet, unlike the Fearbola discourse, this was often an explicit attempt to desecuritize. We can see in this same contestation over the exception, mixed with the politics of expertise yet manifesting in different forms.

Perhaps the difference here lies in the fact that the Ebola outbreak never truly threatened the US in the way that the dominant AUT discourse suggested it could, while COVID-19 ravaged the US. Americans thus watched the terror of Ebola from afar, with very few ever having any personal experience with the horrible disease (or its transmission or the capacity of the US to treat patients). Yet COVID-19 became so ubiquitous that many Americans have either personally suffered through the disease or know someone who has. Moreover, it was easily equated with another ubiquitous disease: seasonal influenza. Both kill in the thousands, but they become expected, known, and thus less terrifying.

Ultimately, this may speak to the power of imagination in security. Christian Enemark's (2007, 1; 2017, xvii) description of diseases that are ripe for securitization as "dreaded diseases" is an apt one. Ebola did not threaten most Americans but is a terrible and deadly disease that has received sensationalist depictions over the years. It had become "the disease people around the world love to fear" (David Quammen, quoted in Smith 2014). It taps into the racialized (and racist) outbreak narrative and intersects with the Dark Continent discourse, sitting as the archetype of the disease originating from the deep, dark African jungles that Robert Kaplan (1994) wrote about in *The Coming Anarchy*. It therefore easily sparks an atavistic fear in the population.

Yet in some parts of the population, it also calls to action: the health workers who volunteered to travel across the world to help end the outbreak and those who argued passionately against the racist and dehumanizing depictions they observed in the solipsist demands for travel bans. Indeed, if this book communicates just one thing, it should be that we are never bound by our societies' worst tendencies, nor by the Schmittian heart of security. There are always multiple perspectives, and these can change over time. But we need to be willing to grapple with them and consider the role that we play in securitization and the contestation that occurs within it.

Notes

Chapter 1

1. A notable exception can be found in Lo 2015.

2. See Buzan et al. 1998 for the most definitive statement.

3. See, for instance, the recent contributions by Rita Floyd (2016, 2019), who argues that the audience is relatively unimportant for securitization.

4. They use an illustrative example of Lene Hansen, who has explicitly offered a poststructuralist expansion of securitization yet also could be associated with other groups for her emphasis on practice. We might also consider figures such as Holger Stritzel (2007, 2014) and Mark Salter (2008b), who have both meshed discursive approaches with frameworks that might be considered sociological.

5. Externalist and internalist readings of context is a distinction offered by Balzacq (2010) but also frequently adopted by those explicitly adopting his "sociological variant of securitization" (see Balzacq et al. 2015, 504).

6. With the latter, as Andrew W. Neal (2019, 71–76) has pointed out, there are different readings of Foucault and his work within critical security studies, with one approach focusing on his methodological work (discourses, dispositifs, problematization) and another focusing on one particular problematization: governmentality.

Chapter 2

1. Critical discourse analysis is used by some as interchangeable with discourse analysis. Yet, as Stritzel (2014, 44), describes it, critical discourse analysis provides far more emphasis on the embeddedness of discourse within social practices (including power dynamics, institutions, and resource struggles), to the point of discourse being "ultimately *subordinate*" to them. I do not conceptualize discourse as subordinate to social practices, but instead see the two as mutually constitutive.

Chapter 4

1. To emphasize the repeated nature of such a claim, also note Sanjay Gupta in Newsroom 2014c; Carol Costello in Newsroom 2014d; Chris Wallace in FNS 2014a; Matt Lauer in Today 2014a; David Gregory in MTP 2014a.

2. See Achenbach 2014; Bump 2014a; Caplan 2014; Kristof 2014a for uses of this tweet to criticize the AUT discourse.

3. Again, numerous examples of this representation are apparent. See Carter and Hanna 2014; Fahrenthold 2014; McCoy 2014d; Root Wolpe 2014.

4. See Klein 2014; Nakamura 2014a; Strain 2014; Sun and Eilperin 2014 for quotes.

5. These included, but were not limited to: Ebola Prevention Act 2014; Keeping America Safe from Ebola Act 2014; Stop Ebola Act 2014.

Chapter 5

1. I have written on this in more theoretical detail elsewhere. See Kirk 2020.

Chapter 6

1. In one notable case, a doctor who walked through Hartsfield-Jackson Atlanta International Airport in a hazmat suit with "CDC is lying" written on the back was interviewed by CNN, Fox News, and USA Today. Each emphasized his position as a medical doctor.

2. Notable exceptions include the work of Adam Nossiter (2014c, 2014d; Nossiter and Solomon 2014).

3. The similarity between the media depictions of Huanan Seafood Market during COVID-19 and those of the "primitive farms" of Guangdong during the SARS epidemic that Wald (2008, 5–7) discusses is striking.

References

ABC News. 2014. "From Coffee Stand to Bowling Alley: Retracing Steps of Doctor Who Tested Positive for Ebola." October 25, 2014. https://abcnews.go.com/Health /retracing-steps-dr-craig-spencer-ebola-diagnosis/story?id=26418093

Abeysinghe, Sudeepa. 2016. "Ebola at the Borders: Newspaper Representations and the Politics of Border Control." *Third World Quarterly* 37, no. 3: 452–467.

Abraham, Thomas. 2011. "The Chronicle of a Disease Foretold: Pandemic H1N1 and the Construction of a Global Health Threat." *Political Studies* 59, no. 4: 797–812.

Abrahamsen, Rita. 2005. "Blair's Africa: The Politics of Securitization and Fear." *Alternatives: Global, Local, Political* 30, no. 1: 55–80.

Abrahamsen, Rita and Michael C. Williams. 2009. "Security Beyond the State: Global Security Assemblages in International Politics." *International Political Sociology* 3, no. 1: 1–17.

Abutaleb, Yasmeen, Philip Rucker, Josh Dawsey, and Robert Costa. 2020. "Trump's Den of Dissent: Inside the White House Task Force as Coronavirus Surges." *Washington Post*, October 19, 2020. https://www.washingtonpost.com/politics/trumps-den -of-dissent-inside-the-white-house-task-force-as-coronavirus-surges/2020/10/19/7ff8 ee6a-0a6e-11eb-859b-f9c27abe638d_story.html

Achenbach, Joel. 2014. "Hiccups Could Mean Ebola!" *Washington Post*, August 5, 2014. Retrieved from Factiva database.

Achenbach, Joel and Brady Dennis. 2014. "Contagion of Fear." *Washington Post*, October 19, 2014. Retrieved from Factiva database.

Aginam, Obijiofor. 2005. *Global Health Governance: International Law and Public Health in a Divided World*. Toronto: University of Toronto Press.

Alcabes, Phillip. 2009. *Dread: How Fear and Fantasy Have Fueled Epidemics from the Black Death to the Avian Flu*. New York: Public Affairs.

Aldis, William. 2008. "Health Security as a Public Health Concept." *Health Policy and Planning* 23, no. 6: 369–375.

All In with Chris Hayes (All In). 2014a. Broadcast transcript. *MSNBC*, August 4, 2014. Retrieved from Factiva database.

All In. 2014b. Broadcast transcript. *MSNBC*, November 11, 2014. Retrieved from Factiva database.

Altman, Drew. 2020. "Understanding the US Failure on Coronavirus." *BMJ* 370 (m3417): 1–3.

Amoore, Louise. 2006. "Biometric Borders: Governing Mobilities in the War on Terror." *Political Geography* 25, no. 3: 336–351.

Amoore, Louise and Marieke de Goede. 2005. "Governance, Risk and Dataveillance in the War on Terror." *Crime, Law, and Social Change* 43, no. 2: 149–173.

Amoore, Louise and Marieke de Goede. 2008. "Transactions after 9/11: The Banal Face of the Preemptive Strike." *Transactions of the Institute of British Geographers* 33, no. 2: 173–185.

Anderson Cooper 360 (AC360). 2014a. Broadcast transcript. *CNN*, August 4, 2014. Retrieved from Factiva database.

AC360. 2014b. Broadcast transcript. *CNN*, August 5, 2014. Retrieved from Factiva database.

AC360. 2014c. Broadcast transcript. *CNN*, August 26, 2014. Retrieved from Factiva database.

AC360. 2014d. Broadcast transcript. *CNN*, September 18, 2014. Retrieved from Factiva database.

AC360. 2014e. Broadcast transcript. *CNN*, October 24, 2014. Retrieved from Factiva database.

Aradau, Claudia. 2004. "Security and the Democratic Scene: Desecuritization and Emancipation." *Journal of International Relations and Development* 7, no. 4: 388–413.

Aradau, Claudia. 2008. *Rethinking Trafficking in Women: Politics out of Security*. Basingstroke, UK: Palgrave Macmillian.

Aradau, Claudia, Luis Lobo-Guerrero, and Rens van Munster. 2008. "Security, Technologies of Risk, and the Political." *Security Dialogue* 39, no. 2–3: 147–154.

Aradau, Claudia and Rens van Munster. 2008. "Governing Terrorism Through Risk: Taking Precautions, (Un)Knowing the Future." *European Journal of International Relations* 13, no. 1: 89–115.

Aradau, Claudia and Rens van Munster. 2009. "Exceptionalism and the War on Terror: Criminology meets International Relations." *The British Journal of Criminology* 49, no. 5: 686–701.

Aradau, Claudia and Rens van Munster. 2011. *Politics of Catastrophe: Genealogies of the Unknown*. London: Routledge.

Arendt, Hannah. 1958. *The Human Condition*. Chicago: University of Chicago Press.

Attiah, Karen. 2014. "The World Is Still Far from the Finish Line on Ebola." *Washington Post*, November 6, 2014. Retrieved from Factiva database.

Balzacq, Thierry. 2005. "The Three Faces of Securitization: Political Agency, Audience, and Context." *European Journal of International Relations* 11, no. 2: 171–201.

Balzacq, Thierry. 2010. "A Theory of Securitization: Origins, Core Assumptions, and Variants." In *Securitization Theory: How Security Problems Emerge and Dissolve*, edited by Thierry Balzacq, 1–30. Abingdon, UK: Routledge.

Balzacq, Thierry. 2019. "Securitization Theory: Past, Present, and Future." *Polity* 51, no. 2: 331–348.

Balzacq, Thierry, Sarah Léonard, and Jan Ruzicka. 2015. "Securitization Revisited: Theory and Cases." *International Relations* 30, no. 4: 494–531.

Ban, Ki-Moon. 2014. "The Ebola Fight is Far From Over." *Washington Post*, November 8, 2014. Retrieved from Factiva database.

Barnett, Tony and Gwyn Prins. 2006. "HIV/AIDS and Security: Fact, Fiction and Evidence: A Report to UNAIDS." *International Affairs* 82, no. 2: 359–368.

Beck, Ulrich. 2002. "The Terrorist Threat: World Risk Society Revisited." *Theory, Culture & Society* 19, no. 4: 39–55.

Benedetto, Richard. 2014. "Rookie Senators, Beware: Obama's Failures of Competence Mean Experience Is Back in Vogue." *USA Today*, November 5, 2014. Retrieved from Factiva database.

Benton, Adia. 2017. "Whose Security? Militarization and Securitization during West Africa's Ebola Outbreak." In *The Politics of Fear: Médecins Sans Frontières and the West African Ebola Epidemic*, edited by Michel Hofman and Sokhieng Au, 25–59. New York: Oxford University Press.

Benton, Adia and Kim Yi Dionne. 2014. "Pundits Panicking about Ebola Hurt Cause They Mean to Help." *Washington Post*, September 1, 2014. Retrieved from Factiva database.

Berents, Helen. 2019. "Apprehending the 'Telegenic Dead': Considering Images of Dead Children in Global Politics." *International Political Sociology* 13, no. 2: 145–160.

Berezow, Alex. 2014. "CDC Caught in Ebola Catch-22." *USA Today*, October 24, 2014. Retrieved from Factiva database.

Berlinguer, Giovanni. 2003. "Bioethics, Human Security, and Global Health." In *Global Health Challenges for Human Security*, edited by Lincoln Chen, Jennifer Leaning, and Vasant Narasimhan. Cambridge, MA: Harvard University Press.

Berman, Mark and Amy Ellis Nutt. 2014. "Infected Man Was Allowed to Leave Dallas Hospital." *Washington Post*, October 2, 2014. Retrieved from Factiva database.

Bernstein, Lenny. 2014. "Out of Options, the Dying Sit and Wait." *Washington Post*, September 14, 2014. Retrieved from Factiva database.

Bertrand, Sarah. 2018. "Can the Subaltern Securitize? Postcolonial Perspectives on Securitization Theory and Its Critics." *European Journal of International Security* 3, no. 3: 281–299.

Besser, Richard E. 2014. "Fight Fear of Ebola with the Facts." *Washington Post*, October 15, 2014. Retrieved from Factiva database.

Bigo, Didier. 2002. "Security and Immigration: Toward a Critique of the Governmentality of Unease." *Alternatives: Global, Local, Political* 27, no. 1: 63–92.

Bigo, Didier. 2014. "The (In)Securitization Practices of the Three Universes of EU Border Control: Military/Navy—Border Guards/Police—Database Analysts." *Security Dialogue* 45, no. 3: 209–225.

Bilgin, Pinar. 2011. "The Politics of Studying Securitization? The Copenhagen School in Turkey." *Security Dialogue* 42, no. 4–5: 399–412.

Blake, Aaron. 2014. "Chris Christie Wins Cheers for Ebola Quarantine of Kaci Hickox." *Washington Post.com*, November 7, 2014. Retrieved from Factiva database.

Blow, Charles. 2014. "The Ebola Hysteria." *New York Times*, October 29, 2014. Retrieved from Factiva database.

Booth, Ken. 1997. "Security and Self: Reflection of a Fallen Realist." In *Critical Security Studies: Concepts and Cases*, edited by Keith Krause and Michael C. Williams, 83–119. Minneapolis: University of Minnesota Press.

Booth, Ken. 2007. *Theory of World Security*. Cambridge: Cambridge University Press.

Boyle, Matthew. 2014. "Exclusive—Rand Paul: Obama 'Downplaying' Ebola Threat to America." *Breitbart News*, October 3, 2014. https://www.breitbart.com/politics/2014/10/03/Exclusive-Rand-Paul-Obama-Downplaying-Ebola-Threat-To-America-Travel-Restrictions-Necessary-Because-I-Fear-Potential-Worldwide-Pandemic/.

Bradner, Eric. 2014. "GOP Stokes Border Fears over Ebola, ISIS." *CNN*, October 9, 2014. Retrieved from Factiva database.

Breen, Leah. 2014. "Fighting Ebola, Liberia's 'Invisible Rebel.'" *Washington Post*, August 29, 2014. Retrieved from Factiva database.

Brooks, David and Gail Collins. 2014. "Political Infections." *New York Times* (blog), October 28, 2014. Retrieved from Factiva database.

Brown, DeNeen L. and Abby Phillip. 2014. "Family of Ebola Patient Thomas Eric Duncan Distraught over Death in Dallas." *Washington Post*, October 9, 2014. Retrieved from Factiva database.

Bruni, Frank. 2014. "Republicans, Meet Science." *New York Times*, November 5, 2014. Retrieved from Factiva database.

Bubandt, Nils. 2005. "Vernacular Security: The Politics of Feeling Safe in Global, National and Local Worlds." *Security Dialogue* 36, no. 3: 275–296.

Bump, Philip. 2014a. "The Ebola Epidemic Has Infected America's Political Debate, If Nothing Else." *Washington Post*, August 6, 2014. Retrieved from Factiva database.

Bump, Philip. 2014b. "The Main Thing on Voters' Minds Heading into Election Day Might Have Been Ebola." *Washington Post*, November 7, 2014. Retrieved from Factiva database.

Bump, Philip. 2020. "The Self-Anointed 'Wartime President' Finds a New, More Exciting War." *Washington Post*, June 1, 2020. https://www.washingtonpost.com /politics/2020/06/01/self-anointed-wartime-president-finds-new-more-exciting-war/.

Burci, Gian Luca. 2014. "Ebola, the Security Council and the Securitization of Public Health." *Questions of International Law*, December 23, 20214. http://www.qil-qdi.org/ ebola-security-council-securitization-public-health/

Butler, Judith. 1990. *Gender Trouble: Feminism and the Subversion of Identity*. New York: Routledge.

Buzan, Barry, Ole Wæver, and Jaap de Wilde. 1998. *Security: A New Framework for Analysis*. Boulder, CO: Lynne Rienner.

Buzan, Barry and Ole Wæver. 2009. "Macrosecuritization and Security Constellations: Reconsidering Scale in Securitization Theory." *Review of International Studies* 35, no. 2: 253–276.

Caballero-Anthony, Mely. 2006. "Combating Infectious Disease in East Asia: Securitization and Global Public Goods for Health and Human Security." *Journal of International Affairs* 59, no. 2: 105–127.

Campbell, David. 1998. *Writing Security: United States Foreign Policy and the Politics of Identity*. Minneapolis: University of Minnesota.

Caplan, Arthur L. 2014. "Why Do Two White Americans Get the Ebola Serum While Hundreds of Africans Die?" *Washington Post*, August 6, 2014. Retrieved from Factiva database.

Caremel, Jean-François, Sylvain Landry B. Faye, and Ramatou Ouedraogo. 2017. "The 'Humanitarian' Response to the Ebola Epidemic in Guinea." In *The Politics of Fear: Médecins Sans Frontières and the West African Ebola Epidemic*, edited by Michel Hofman and Sokhieng Au, 63–80. New York: Oxford University Press.

Carey, Benedict. 2014. "Ebola's Other Contagious Threat: Hysteria." *New York Times*, October 16, 2014. Retrieved from Factiva database.

Carter, Chelsea J. and Jason Hanna. 2014. "U.S. Doctor Treated for Ebola Drawn to Mission Work Since Youth." *CNN*, August 2, 2014. Retrieved from Factiva database.

Caso, Federica. 2020. "Are We at War? The Rhetoric of War in the Coronavirus Pandemic." *The Disorder of Things*, April 10, 2020. https://thedisorderofthings.com/2020/04/10/are-we-at-war-the-rhetoric-of-war-in-the-coronavirus-pandemic/.

CBS News. 2014. "What We Know About Ebola Patient Dr. Craig Spencer's Movements." October 24, 2014. https://www.cbsnews.com/news/ebola-outbreak-what-we-know-about-patient-dr-craig-spencers-movements/.

Centers for Disease Control and Prevention (CDC). 2014a. "CDC Press Conference: CDC Confirms First Ebola Case Diagnosed in the United States." CDC Newsroom Releases. September 30, 2014. https://www.cdc.gov/media/releases/2014/t0930-ebola-confirmed-case.html.

CDC. 2014b. "Enhanced Ebola Screening to Start at Five U.S. Airports and New Tracking Program for all People Entering U.S. from Ebola-affected Countries." CDC Newsroom Releases. October 8, 2014. https://www.cdc.gov/media/releases/2014/p1008-ebola-screening.html.

CDC. 2014c. "CDC Update on Ebola Response, 10-13-2014." CDC Newsroom Releases. October 10, 2014. https://www.cdc.gov/media/releases/2014/t1013-ebola-reponse-update.html.

CDC. 2014d. "CDC Tightened Guidance for U.S. Healthcare Workers on Personal Protective Equipment for Ebola." CDC Newsroom Releases. October 20, 2014. https://www.cdc.gov/media/releases/2014/fs1020-ebola-personal-protective-equipment.html.

Chapman, Audrey. 2016. *Global Health, Human Rights, and the Challenge of Neoliberal Policies.* Cambridge: Cambridge University Press.

Chen, David W. 2014. "A Tepid Thumbs Up Is the Best Many Can Muster for Cuomo." *New York Times*, November 3, 2014. Retrieved from Factiva database.

Chen, Lincoln and Vasant Narasimhan. 2003. "A Human Security Agenda for Global Health." In *Global Health Challenges for Human Security*, edited by Lincoln Chen, Jennifer Leaning, and Vasant Narasimhan. Cambridge, MA: Harvard University Press.

Christensen, Jen. 2014. "Ebola Is Here: 5 Reasons Not to Panic." *CNN*, August 5, 2014. Retrieved from Factiva database.

Ciută, Felix. 2009. "Security and the Problem of Context: A Hermeneutical Critique of Securitization Theory." *Review of International Studies* 35, no. 2: 301–326.

CNN. 2014a. "New Hampshire Senate Debate." Broadcast transcript. October 25, 2014. Retrieved from Factiva database.

CNN. 2014b. "Live Coverage of Midterm Election Results." Broadcast transcript. November 4, 2014. Retrieved from Factiva database.

Cohen, Elizabeth. 2014. "Ebola in the Air? A Nightmare That Could Happen." *CNN*, September 12, 2014. Retrieved from Factiva database.

Collier, Stephen J. and Andrew Lakoff. 2008. "The Problem of Securing Health." In *Biosecurity Interventions: Global Health and Security in Question*, edited by Andrew Lakoff and Stephen J. Collier, 7–32. New York: Columbia University Press.

Committee on Energy and Commerce (CEC). 2014a. *Examining the US Public Health Response to the Ebola Outbreak. Hearing before the Subcommittee on Oversight and Investigation.* 113th Congress.

CEC. 2014b. *Update on the US Public Health Response to the Ebola Outbreak. Hearing before the Subcommittee on Oversight and Investigations.* 113th Congress.

Committee on Health, Education, Labor, and Pensions (CHELP). 2014. *Ebola in West Africa: A Global Challenge and Public Health Threat. Joint Hearing before the Committee on Health, Education, Labor, and Pensions and Subcommittee on Labor, Health and Human Services, Education and Related Agencies of the Committee on Appropriations,* 113th Congress.

Committee on Foreign Affairs (CFA), House of Representatives. 2014a. *Combating the Ebola Threat: Hearing before the Subcommittee on Africa, Global Health, Global Human Rights, and International Organizations.* 113th Congress.

CFA. 2014b. *Global Efforts to Fight Ebola: Hearing before the Subcommittee on Africa, Global Health, Global Human Rights, and International Organizations.* 113th Congress.

CFA. 2014c. *Fighting Ebola: A Ground-Level View. Hearing before the Subcommittee on Africa, Global Health, Global Human Rights, and International Organizations.* 113th Congress.

Committee on Homeland Security (CHS). 2014. *Ebola in the Homeland: The Importance of Effective International, Federal, State, and Local Coordination. Field Hearing before the Committee on Homeland Security, House of Representatives.* 113th Congress.

Condon, George E. Jr. 2015. "Obama's Ebola Victory Lap." *Atlantic*, February 11, 2015. https://www.theatlantic.com/politics/archive/2015/02/obamas-ebola-victory-lap /442554/.

Coons, Chris. 2015. *Letter to the Department of Defense re: Ebola*. January 7, 2015. https://www.coons.senate.gov/imo/media/doc/Sen.%20Coons%20letter%20to%20 DoD%20re.%20Ebola.pdf.

Corry, Olaf. 2012. "Securitization and 'Riskification': Second-order Security and the Politics of Climate Change." *Millennium: Journal of International Studies* 40, no. 2: 235–258.

Côté, Adam. 2016. "Agents without Agency: Assessing the Role of the Audience in Securitization Theory." *Security Dialogue* 47, no. 6: 541–558.

Coulter, Ann. 2014. "Ebola Doc's Condition Downgraded to 'Idiotic.'" Ann Coulter (website). August 6, 2014. http://www.anncoulter.com/columns/2014-08-06.html.

Cruz, Ted. 2014a. "Ban Flights from Ebola-Stricken Nations." *TribTalk*, October 15, 2014. http://www.tribtalk.org/2014/10/15/ban-flights-from-ebola-stricken-nations/.

Cruz, Ted. 2014b. "Sen. Cruz: Arguments against a Flight Ban to Prevent Ebola Spread Don't Make Sense." Press Release. US Senator for Texas Ted Cruz (website). October 19, 2014. http://www.cruz.senate.gov/?p=press_release&id=1815.

CSIS Science and Technical Committee and Panel on Crisis Management (CSIS). 1984. *America's Hidden Vulnerabilities: Crisis Management in a Society of Networks*. Washington, DC: Center for Strategic and International Studies, Georgetown University.

Curley, Melissa and Jonathon Herington. 2011. "The Securitization of Avian Influenza: International Discourses and Domestic Politics in Asia." *Review of International Studies* 37, no. 1: 141–166.

Daigal, David. 2014. "Inside the Ebola Outbreak with the CDC." *CNN*, August 13, 2014. Retrieved from Factiva database.

Dausey, David J. 2014. "Naïve Optimism Won't Protect You from Ebola." *USA Today*, October 2, 2014. Retrieved from Factiva database.

Davies, Sara E. 2008. "Securitizing Infectious Disease." *International Affairs* 84, no. 2: 295–313.

Davies, Sara E. 2010. *Global Politics of Health*. Cambridge: Polity.

Davies, Sara E. 2014. "Internet Surveillance and Disease Outbreaks." In the *Routledge Handbook of Global Health Security*, edited by Simon Rushton and Jeremy Youde, 226–238. Abingdon, UK: Routledge.

Davies, Sara E. and Belinda Bennett. 2016. "A Gendered Human Rights Analysis of Ebola and Zika: Locating Gender in Global Health Emergencies." *International Affairs* 92, no. 5: 1041–1060.

Davies, Sara E., Adam Kamradt-Scott, and Simon Rushton. 2015. *Disease Diplomacy: International Norms and Global Health Security*. Baltimore: Johns Hopkins University Press.

De Goede, Marieke. 2008. "Beyond Risk: Premediation and the Post-9/11 Security Imagination." *Security Dialogue* 39, no. 2–3: 155–176.

De Goede, Marieke and Beatrice de Graaf. 2013. "Sentencing Risk: Temporality and Precaution in Terrorism Trials." *International Political Sociology* 7, no. 3: 313–331.

de Waal, Alex. 2014. "Militarizing Global Health." *Boston Review*, November 11, 2014. http://bostonreview.net/world/alex-de-waal-militarizing-global-health-ebola.

DeLaet, Debra L. 2014. "Whose Interests Is the Securitization of Health Serving?" In *Routledge Handbook of Global Health Security*, edited by Simon Rushton and Jeremy Youde, 339–348. Abingdon, UK: Routledge.

Deloffre, Maryam Zarnegar. 2014. "Will AFRICOM's Ebola Response Be Watershed Moment for International Action on Human Security?" *Washington Post*, September 29, 2014. Retrieved from Factiva database.

Department of Defense (DoD). 2014. "Department of Defense Press Briefing by Rear Adm. Kirby in the Pentagon Briefing Room." Press briefing transcript. August 5, 2014. https://www.defense.gov/Newsroom/Transcripts/Transcript/Article/606902/depart ment-of-defense-press-briefing-by-rear-adm-kirby-in-the-pentagon-briefing/.

Dionne, Kim Yi. 2014. "Ebola Experimental Treatment Only for the Exceptional." *Washington Post*, August 11, 2014. Retrieved from Factiva database.

Doty, Roxanne Lynn. 1996. *Imperial Encounters*. Minneapolis: University of Minnesota Press.

Doty, Roxanne Lynn. 1998. "Immigration and the Politics of Security." *Security Studies* 8, no. 2–3: 71–93.

Doty, Roxanne Lynn. 2007. "States of Exception on the Mexico–U.S. Border: Security, 'Decisions,' and Civilian Border Patrols." *International Political Sociology* 1, no. 2: 113–137.

Drezner, Daniel W. 2014a. "Scare-Mongering about Ebola Is Not Such a Great Idea." *Washington Post*, August 15, 2014. Retrieved from Factiva database.

Drezner, Daniel W. 2014b. "Seven Things We Now Know about How the World Has Handled Ebola." *Washington Post*, October 6, 2014. Retrieved from Factiva database.

Drezner, Daniel W. 2014c. "The First Rule of Ebola Security Theater Is That You Can't Admit It's Ebola Security Theater." *Washington Post*, October 28, 2014. Retrieved from Factiva database.

Dunn, Kevin C. and Iver B. Neumann. 2016. *Undertaking Discourse Analysis for Social Research*. Ann Arbor: University of Michigan Press.

Dunne, Tim and Nicholas J. Wheeler. 2004. "We the Peoples: Contending Discourses of Security in Human Rights Theory and Practice." *International Relations* 18, no.1: 9–24.

Dupont, Alan. 2001. *HIV/AIDS: A Major International Security Issue*. Canberra: Australian Aid Program.

Early Start. 2014a. Broadcast transcript. *CNN*, August 26, 2014. Retrieved from Factiva database.

Early Start. 2014b. Broadcast transcript. *CNN*, September 25, 2014. Retrieved from Factiva database.

Early Start. 2014c. Broadcast transcript. *CNN*, October 1, 2014. Retrieved from Factiva database.

Early Start. 2014d. Broadcast transcript. *CNN*, October 24, 2014. Retrieved from Factiva database.

Early Start. 2014e. Broadcast transcript. *CNN*, November 7, 2014. Retrieved from Factiva database.

Ebola Prevention Act. 2014. H.R. 5692. 113th Congress. Retrieved from https://www.congress.gov/bill/113th-congress/house-bill/5692.

Edkins, Jenny. 2002. "After the Subject of International Security." In *Politics and Post-Structuralism*, edited by Alan Finlayson and Jeremy Valentine, 66–82. Edinburgh: Edinburgh University Press.

Eilperin, Juliet. 2014a. "President Grapples with Health and Political Challenges." *Washington Post*, October 17, 2014. Retrieved from Factiva database.

Eilperin, Juliet. 2014b. "Obama May Appoint an Ebola Czar, He Says." *Washington Post*, October 17, 2014. Retrieved from Factiva database.

Eilperin, Juliet and David Nakamura. 2014. "Obama Taps Ron Klain as Ebola Czar." *Washington Post*, October 18, 2014. Retrieved from Factiva database.

Ejdus, Filip and Mina Božović. 2017. "Grammar, Context and Power: Securitization of the 2010 Belgrade Pride Parade." *Southeast European and Black Sea Studies* 17, no. 1: 17–34.

Elbe, Stefan. 2002. "HIV/AIDS and the Changing Landscape of War in Africa." *International Security* 27, no. 2: 159–177.

Elbe, Stefan. 2005. "AIDS, Security, Biopolitics." *International Relations* 19, no. 4: 403–419.

Elbe, Stefan. 2006. "Should HIV/AIDS Be Securitized? The Ethical Dilemmas of Linking HIV/AIDS and Security." *International Studies Quarterly* 50, no. 1: 119–144.

Elbe, Stefan. 2008. "Risking Lives: AIDS, Security, and Three Concepts of Risk." *Security Dialogue* 39, no. 2–3: 177–198.

Elbe, Stefan. 2009. *Virus Alert: Security, Governmentality, and the Aids Pandemic*. New York: Columbia University Press.

Elbe, Stefan. 2010. "Haggling over Viruses: The Downside Risks of Securitizing Infectious Disease." *Health Policy and Planning* 25, no. 6: 476–485.

Elbe, Stefan. 2014. "The Pharmaceuticalisation of Security: Molecular Biomedicine, Antiviral Stockpiles, and Global Health Security." *Review of International Studies* 40, no. 5: 919–938.

Elbe, Stefan. 2018. *Pandemics, Pills, and Politics: Governing Global Health Security*. Baltimore: Johns Hopkins University Press.

Elbe, Stefan. 2021. "Bioinformational Diplomacy: Global Health Emergencies, Data Sharing, and Sequential Life." *European Journal of International Relations* 27, no. 3: 657–681.

Enemark, Christian. 2007. *Disease and Security: Natural Plagues and Biological Weapons in East Asia*. London: Routledge.

Enemark, Christian. 2009. "Is Pandemic Flu a Security Threat?" *Survival* 51, no. 1: 191–214.

Enemark, Christian. 2017a. "Ebola, Disease-Control, and the Security Council: From Securitization to Securing Circulation." *Journal of Global Security Studies* 2, no. 2: 137–149.

Enemark, Christian. 2017b. *Biosecurity Dilemmas: Dreaded Diseases, Ethical Responses, and the Health of Nations*. Washington, DC: Georgetown University Press.

Ericson, Richard and Aaron Doyle. 2004. "Catastrophic Risk, Insurance, and Terrorism." *Economy and Society* 33, no. 2: 135–173.

Erin Burnett: Outfront (EB:O). 2014a. Broadcast transcript. *CNN*, April 7, 2014. Retrieved from Factiva database.

EB:O. 2014b. Broadcast transcript. *CNN*, April 15, 2014. Retrieved from Factiva database.

EB:O. 2014c. Broadcast transcript. *CNN*, July 31, 2014. Retrieved from Factiva database.

EB:O. 2014d. Broadcast transcript. *CNN*, August 1, 2014. Retrieved from Factiva database.

EB:O. 2014e. Broadcast transcript. *CNN*, August 4, 2014. Retrieved from Factiva database.

EB:O. 2014f. Broadcast transcript. *CNN*, October 24, 2014. Retrieved from Factiva database.

Eskew, Carter. 2014. "Dems Off the 'Mark.'" *Washington Post*, November 5, 2014. Retrieved from Factiva database.

Ewald, François. 2002. "The Return of Descartes' Malicious Demon: An Outline of a Philosophy of Precaution." In *Embracing Risk: The Changing Culture of Insurance and Responsibility*, editors Tom Baker and Jonathan Simon, 273–301. Chicago: University of Chicago Press.

Eyal, Gil. 2019. *The Crisis of Expertise*. Cambridge: Polity.

Fahrenthold, David A. 2014. "Doctor with Ebola Arrives in Atlanta to Receive Treatment." *Washington Post*, August 3, 2014. Retrieved from Factiva database.

Fareed Zakaria GPS. 2014. Broadcast transcript. *CNN*, August 3, 2014. Retrieved from Factiva database.

Farhi, Paul. 2014. Ebola Coverage: Overtime, but Not Necessarily Overboard. *Washington Post*, October 6, 2014. Retrieved from Factiva database.

Farmer, Paul. 2005. *Pathologies of Power: Health, Human Rights, and the New War on the Poor*. Berkeley: University of California Press.

Fearnley, Lyle. 2008. "Redesigning Syndromic Surveillance for Biosecurity." In *Biosecurity Interventions: Global Health and Security in Question*, edited by Andrew Lakoff and Stephen J. Collier, 61–88. New York: Columbia University Press.

Ferhani, Adam, and Simon Rushton. 2020. "The International Health Regulations, COVID-19, and Bordering Practices: Who Gets In, What Gets Out, and Who Gets Rescued?" *Contemporary Security Policy* 41, no. 3: 458–477.

Fidler, David P. 2015. "Epic Failure of Ebola and Global Health Security." *Brown Journal of World Affairs* 21, no. 2: 180–198.

Fink, Sheri. 2014a. "With Aid Doctors Gone, Ebola Fight Grows Harder." *New York Times*, August 17, 2014. Retrieved from Factiva database.

Fink, Sheri. 2014b. "Life, Death and Careful Routine Fill the Day at a Liberian Clinic." *New York Times*, October 8, 2014. Retrieved from Factiva database.

Fink, Sheri. 2014c. "In Layers of Gear, Offering Healing Hand to Ebola Patients in Liberia." *New York Times*, October 17, 2014. Retrieved from Factiva database.

Fink, Sheri. 2014d. "Improvising on Ebola's Front Lines." *New York Times*, October 27, 2014. Retrieved from Factiva database.

Fink, Sheri. 2014e. "The Capricious Hand of Ebola: One Boy Survives as Others Die." *New York Times*, November 10, 2014. Retrieved from Factiva database.

Fisher, Marc. 2014. "At the Polls, Voters Express Exasperation and Anxiety." *Washington Post*, November 5, 2014. Retrieved from Factiva database.

The Five. 2014a. Broadcast transcript. *Fox News*, September 16, 2014. Retrieved from Factiva database.

The Five. 2014b. Broadcast transcript. *Fox News*, September 30, 2014. Retrieved from Factiva database.

The Five. 2014c. Broadcast transcript. *Fox News*, October 27, 2014. Retrieved from Factiva database.

Flanagin, Jake. 2014a. "How Environmentalism Can Stop Ebola." *New York Times* (blog), July 17, 2014. Retrieved from Factiva database.

Flanagin, Jake. 2014b. "What Happens to the News When Ebola Reaches New York." *New York Times* (blog), October 28, 2014. Retrieved from Factiva database.

Floyd, Rita. 2016. "Extraordinary or Ordinary Emergency Measures: What, and Who, Defines the Success of Securitization?" *Cambridge Review of International Affairs* 29, no. 2: 677–694.

Floyd, Rita. 2019. *The Morality of Security: A Theory of Just Securitization*. Cambridge: Cambridge University Press.

Flynn, Gerard and Susan Scutti. 2014. "Smuggled Bushmeat is Ebola's Back Door to America." *Newsweek*, August 21, 2014. http://www.newsweek.com/2014/08/29 /smuggled-bushmeat-ebolas-back-door-america-265668.html.

Foege, William, James Mason, and David Satcher. 2014. "Why U.S. Must Lead Ebola Fight." *USA Today*, September 5, 2014. Retrieved from Factiva database.

Foucault, Michel. 1976. *Society Must Be Defended: Lectures at the Collège de France 1975–76*, translated by David Macy. New York: Picador.

Foucault, Michel. 1977. *Discipline and Punish: The Birth of the Prison*, translated by A. Sheridan. New York: Pantheon.

Foucault, Michel. 1980. *Power/Knowledge: Selected Interviews and Other Writings*, translated by Colin Gordon. New York: Pantheon Books.

Fox News. 2014. "Huckabee: Ebola Scare Reveals Public's Lack of Faith in Gov't." October 5, 2014. https://insider.foxnews.com/2014/10/05/mike-huckabee-ebola-scare -reveals-publics-lack-faith-govt.

Fox News Sunday (FNS). 2014a. Broadcast transcript. *Fox News*, August 3, 2014. Retrieved from Factiva database.

FNS. 2014b. Broadcast transcript. *Fox News*, October 19, 2014. Retrieved from Factiva database.

FNS. 2014c. Broadcast transcript. *Fox News*, October 26, 2014. Retrieved from Factiva database.

FNS. 2014d. Broadcast transcript. *Fox News*, November 2, 2014. Retrieved from Factiva database.

Garamone, Jim. 2014. "Kelly: Southcom Keeps Watch on Ebola Situation." Article. US Department of Defense (website). October 8, 2014. https://www.defense.gov /Explore/News/Article/Article/603408/.

Garrett, Laurie. 2014a. "Opinion: Why Ebola Epidemic Is Spinning Out of Control." *CNN*, July 24, 2014. https://edition.cnn.com/2014/07/24/opinion/garrett-ebola /index.html.

Garrett, Laurie. 2014b. "You Are Not Nearly Scared Enough About Ebola." *Foreign Policy*, August 15, 2014. http://foreignpolicy.com/2014/08/15/you-are-not-nearly -scared-enough-about-ebola/.

Gasper, Des. 2005. "Securing Humanity: Situating 'Human Security' as Concept and Discourse." *Journal of Human Development* 6, no. 2: 221–245.

Gatherer, Derek. 2014. "What Happens to Your Body If You Get Ebola?" *The Conversation*, June 17, 2014. https://theconversation.com/what-happens-to-your-body-if -you-get-ebola-28116.

Gerson, Michael. 2014a. "Bet on Africa Rising; The Diverse Continent Has Fast-Growing Economies and Stable Nations." *Washington Post*, August 5, 2014. Retrieved from Factiva database.

Gerson, Michael. 2014b. "Ebola Fever." *Washington Post*, August 8, 2014. Retrieved from Factiva database.

Gerson, Michael. 2014c. "The Ebola Crisis Demands That America Act." *Washington Post*, September 5, 2014. Retrieved from Factiva database.

Gerson, Michael. 2014d. "Ethical Choices Surround a Potential Ebola Vaccine." *Washington Post*, October 7, 2014. Retrieved from Factiva database.

Gettleman, Jeffrey. 2014. "Ebola Should Be Easy to Treat." *New York Times*, December 21, 2014. Retrieved from Factiva database.

Ghebreyesus, Tedros Adhanom. 2017. "All Roads Lead to Universal Health Coverage." Commentaries. *World Health Organization*, July 17, 2017. https://www.who.int /news-room/commentaries/detail/all-roads-lead-to-universal-health-coverage.

Gladstone, Rick. 2014. "New Concerns Over Response to Ebola Crisis." *New York Times*, December 3, 2014. Retrieved from Factiva database.

Gostin, Lawrence O. 2014. *Global Health Law*. Cambridge, MA: Harvard University Press.

Gozdecka, Dorota Anna. 2021. "Human Rights During the Pandemic: COVID-19 and the Securitization of Health." *Nordic Journal of Human Rights* 39, no. 3: 205–223.

Graham, Frankin. 2014. "Thank God for Saved Ebola Doc; Curing Kent Brantly Was No Dilemma. Comfy Ethicists Need Dose of Reality." *USA Today*, August 22, 2104. Retrieved from Factiva database.

Gray, Harriet and Anja K. Franck. 2019. "Refugees As/at Risk: The Gendered and Racialized Underpinnings of Securitization in British Media Narratives." *Security Dialogue* 50, no. 3: 275–291.

On the Record with Greta (Greta). 2014a. Broadcast transcript. *Fox News*, August 6, 2014. Retrieved from Factiva database.

Greta. 2014b. Broadcast transcript. *Fox News*, October 13, 2014. Retrieved from Factiva database.

Greta. 2014b. Broadcast transcript. *Fox News*, October 27, 2014. Retrieved from Factiva database.

Guevara, Maria S. 2022. "A Humanitarian Perspective: Keeping People and Their Health, Not National Security, at the Centre." *Australian Journal of International Affairs* 76, no. 1: 17–21.

Gupta, Sanjay. 2014. "Ebola: A Swift, Effective and Bloody Killer." *CNN*, April 14, 2014. Retrieved from Factiva database.

Hajer, Maarten. 1995. *The Politics of Environmental Discourse: Ecological Modernization and the Policy Process*. Oxford: Clarendon Press.

Hameiri, Shahar. 2014. "Avian Influenza, 'Viral Sovereignty,' and the Politics of Health Security in Indonesia." *Pacific Review* 27, no. 3: 333–356.

Hameiri, Shahar and Lee Jones. 2015. *Governing Borderless Threats: Non-Traditional Security and the Politics of State Transformation*. Cambridge: Cambridge University Press.

Hannity. 2014a. Broadcast transcript. *Fox News*, September 30, 2014. Retrieved from Factiva database.

Hannity. 2014b. Broadcast transcript. *Fox News*, October 7, 2014. Retrieved from Factiva database.

Hannity. 2014c. Broadcast transcript. *Fox News*, October 23, 2014. Retrieved from Factiva database.

Hanrieder, Tine and Christian Kreuder-Sonnen. 2014. "WHO Decides on the Exception? Securitization and Emergency Governance in Global Health." *Security Dialogue* 45, no. 4: 331–348.

Hansen, Lene. 2000. "The Little Mermaid's Silent Security Dilemma and the Absence of Gender in the Copenhagen School." *Millennium: Journal of International Studies* 29, no. 2: 285–306.

Hansen, Lene. 2006. *Security as Practice: Discourse Analysis and the Bosnian War*. New York: Routledge.

Hansen, Lene. 2011. "The Politics of Securitization and the Muhammad Cartoon Crisis: A Post-structuralist Perspective." *Security Dialogue* 42, no. 4–5: 357–369.

Hansen, Lene. 2012. "Reconstructing Desecuritization: The Normative-Political in the Copenhagen School and Directions for How to Apply It." *Review of International Studies* 38, no. 3: 525–546.

Hardball. 2014a. Broadcast transcript. *MSNBC*, September 16, 2014. Retrieved from Factiva database.

Hardball. 2014b. Broadcast transcript. *MSNBC*, October 1, 2014. Retrieved from Factiva database.

Hardball. 2014c. Broadcast transcript. *MSNBC*, October 15, 2014. Retrieved from Factiva database.

Hardball. 2014d. Broadcast transcript. *MSNBC*, October 28, 2014. Retrieved from Factiva database.

Harman, Sophie. 2012. *Global Health Governance*. London: Routledge.

Harman, Sophie. 2016. "Ebola, Gender, and Conspicuously Invisible Women in Global Health Governance." *Third World Quarterly* 37, no. 3: 524–541.

Harman, Sophie and Clare Wenham. 2018. "Governing Ebola: Between Global Health and Medical Humanitarianism." *Globalizations* 15, no. 3: 362–376.

Harman, Sophie and Clare Wenham. 2022. "The UN Security Council and Gender in Health Emergencies: What Comes Next?" *Australian Journal of International Affairs* 76, no. 1: 22–26.

Hassan, Hamdy A. 2022. "The Securitization of COVID-19 in Africa: Socio-Economic and Political Implications." *African Security Review* 31, no. 1: 19–32.

Herington, Jonathan. 2010. "Securitization of Infectious Diseases in Vietnam: The Cases of HIV and Avian Influenza." *Health Policy and Planning* 25, no. 6: 467–475.

Higginbottom, Heather. 2014. "The U.S. Government Response to the Ebola Outbreak: Statement Before the U.S. Senate Committee on Appropriations." US Department of State (website). https://2009-2017.state.gov/s/dmr/remarks/2014/233996.htm.

The Hill. 2014. "List: Lawmakers Backing Travel Ban." October 16, 2014. https://thehill.com/policy/transportation/220964-list-lawmakers-backing-travel-ban.

Hills, Kelly. 2016. "Rejecting Quarantine: A Frozen-in-Time Reaction to Disease." In *Ebola's Message*, edited by Nicholas G. Evans, Tara C. Smith, and Maimuna S. Majumder, 217–231. Cambridge, MA: MIT Press.

Hindmarch, Suzanne. 2016. *Securing Health: HIV and the Limits of Securitization*. London: Routledge.

Hogan, Caelainn. 2014. "'There Is No Such Thing as Ebola'; To Fight Ebola, Doctors Must First Explain It." *Washington Post*, July 18, 2014. Retrieved from Factiva database.

Honig, Bonnie. 2009. *Emergency Politics: Paradox, Law, Democracy*. Princeton: Princeton University Press.

Honigsbaum, Mark. 2017. "Between Securitization and Neglect: Managing Ebola at the Borders of Global Health." *Medical History* 61, no. 2: 270–294.

Horton, Richard. 2017. "Offline: Global Health Security—Smart Strategy or Naïve Tactics?" *The Lancet* 389, no. 10072: 892.

Howell, Alison. 2014. "The Global Politics of Medicine: Beyond Global Health, against Securitization Theory." *Review of International Studies* 40, no. 5: 961–987.

Huysmans, Jef. 1998a. "Security! What Do You Mean? From Concept to Thick Signifier." *European Journal of International Relations* 4, no. 2: 226–255.

Huysmans, Jef. 1998b. "The Question of the Limit: Desecuritization and the Aesthetics of Horror in Political Realism." *Millennium: Journal of International Studies* 27, no. 3: 569–589.

Huysmans, Jef. 2004. "Minding Exceptions: The Politics of Insecurity and Liberal Democracy." *Contemporary Political Theory* 3, no. 3: 321–341.

Huysmans, Jef. 2011. "What's in an Act? On Security Speech Acts and Little Security Nothings." *Security Dialogue* 42, no. 4–5: 371–383.

Huysmans, Jef. 2014. *Security Unbound: Enacting Democratic Limits*. London: Routledge.

Ingram, Alan. 2011. "The Pentagon's HIV/AIDS Programmes: Governmentality, Political Economy, Security." *Geopolitics* 16, no. 3: 655–674.

Jasanoff, Sheila. 2004. "The Idiom of Co-production." In *States of knowledge: the co-production of science and social order*, edited by Sheila Jasanoff, 1–12. London: Routledge.

Jasanoff, Sheila and Hilton R. Simmet. 2017. "No Funeral Bells: Public Reason in a 'Post-truth' Age." *Social Studies of Science* 47, no. 5 (October): 751–770.

Johnson, Ayo. 2014. "Can Sierra Leone's Economy Survive Ebola?" *CNN*, September 16, 2014. Retrieved from Factiva database.

Johnson, Sonali and Claudia Garcia-Moreno. 2003. "Gender, Health, and Security." In *Global Health Challenges for Human Security*, edited by Lincoln Chen, Jennifer Leaning, and Vasant Narasimhan. Cambridge, MA: Harvard University Press.

Joint and Coalition Operational Analysis (JCOA). 2016. *Operation United Assistance: The DOD Response to Ebola in West Africa*. Suffolk, VA: US Department of Defense.

Jones, Lee. 2011. "Beyond Securitization: Explaining the Scope of Security Policy in Southeast Asia." *International Relations of the Asia-Pacific* 11, no. 3: 403–432.

Jones, Bryony. 2014. "Are Myths Making the Ebola Outbreak Worse?" *CNN*, August 20, 2014. Retrieved from Factiva database.

Kamradt-Scott, Adam. 2018. "What Went Wrong? The World Health Organization from Swine Flu to Ebola." In *Political Mistakes and Policy Failures in International Relations*, edited by Andreas Kruck, Kai Oppermann, and Alexander Spencer, 193–215. Cham, Switzerland: Palgrave Macmillan.

Kamradt-Scott, Adam and Colin McInnes. 2012. "The Securitization of Pandemic Influenza: Framing, Security, and Public Policy." *Global Public Health* 7, S2: S95-S110.

Kamradt-Scott, Adam, Sophie Harman, Clare Wenham, and Frank Smith III. 2015. *Saving Lives: The Civil-Military Response to the 2014 Ebola Outbreak in West Africa*. Sydney: University of Sydney.

Kang, Cecilia. 2014. "New York Revises Controversial Policy on Ebola Quarantines amid Pressure." *Washington Post*, October 27, 2014. Retrieved from Factiva database.

Kaplan, Robert D. 1994. "The Coming Anarchy." *Atlantic*, February 1994. https://www.theatlantic.com/magazine/archive/1994/02/the-coming-anarchy/304670/.

Keeping America Safe from Ebola Act. 2014. H.R. 5746. 113th Congress. Retrieved from https://www.congress.gov/bill/113th-congress/house-bill/5746.

Kelle, Alexander. 2007. "Securitization of International Public Health: Implications for Global Health Governance and the Biological Weapons Prohibition Regime." *Global Governance* 13, no. 1: 217–235.

Kelly, Representative Michael (PA). 2014. "Keeping America Safe from Ebola." *Congressional Record—House* 160, no. 11: 16208–16209. Retrieved from Congressional Record Permanent Digital Collection.

Kennedy, David. 2016. *A World of Struggle: How Power, Law, and Expertise Shape Global Political Economy*. Princeton: Princeton University Press.

Kerry, John. 2014. "Remarks on the U.S. Response to Ebola for Members of the Diplomatic Corps." US Department of State (website). October 17, 2014. https://2009-2017.state.gov/secretary/remarks/2014/10/233091.htm.

Kidjo, Angelique. 2014. "Don't Let Ebola Dehumanize Africa." *New York Times*, October 30, 2014. Retrieved from Factiva database.

Killough, Ashley. 2014. "Rand Paul Plays up Ebola Fears." *CNN*, October 2, 2014. https://edition.cnn.com/2014/10/01/politics/rand-paul-ebola/index.html.

Kim, Jim Yong and Paul Farmer. 2014. "What the Ebola Fight Is Missing." *Washington Post*, September 1, 2014. Retrieved from Factiva database.

King, Nicholas B. 2002. "Security, Disease, Commerce: Ideologies of Postcolonial Global Health." *Social Studies of Science* 32, no. 5–6: 763–789.

Kirk, Jessica. 2020. "From Threat to Risk? Exceptionalism and the Logics of Health Security." *International Studies Quarterly* 64, no. 2: 266–276.

Kirk, Jessica and Matt McDonald. 2021. "The Politics of Exceptionalism: Security Representations and COVID-19." *Global Studies Quarterly* 1, no. 3: 1–12.

Klein, Betsy. 2014. "Ebola Is a 'National Security Priority,' Obama Says." *CNN*, September 8, 2014. Retrieved from Factiva database.

Koblentz, Gregory D. 2009. *Living Weapons: Biological Warfare and International Security*. Ithaca: Cornell University Press.

Korte, Gregory and Liz Szabo. 2014. "Obama Sends 3,000 Fights; 'It's Spiraling Out of Control'; Us Troops to Set up Africa Base." *USA Today*, September 17, 2014. Retrieved from Factiva database.

Kraut, Alan. 1995. *Silent Travelers: Germs, Genes, and the "Immigrant Menace."* Baltimore: Johns Hopkins University Press.

Kristeva, Julia. 1980. "Word, Dialogue, and Novel." In L. S. Roudiez (ed.), *Desire in Language: A Semiotic Approach to Literature and Art*. New York: Columbia University Press.

Kristof, Nicholas. 2014a. "Fighting Ebola for Us All." *New York Times*, August 7, 2014. Retrieved from Factiva database.

Kristof, Nicholas. 2014b. "The Ebola Fiasco." *New York Times*, September 25, 2014. Retrieved from Factiva database.

Kristof, Nicholas. 2014c. "How to Defeat Ebola." *New York Times*, October 23, 2014. Retrieved from Factiva database.

Krugman, Paul. 2014. "When Government Succeeds." *New York Times*, November 17, 2014. Retrieved from Factiva database.

Labonte, Ronald and Michelle L. Gagnon. 2010. "Framing Health and Foreign Policy: Lessons for Global Health Diplomacy." *Globalization and Health* 6, no. 1: 14–33.

Laclau, Ernesto and Chantal Mouffe. 1985. *Hegemony and Socialist Strategy: Towards a Radical Democratic Politics*. London: Verso.

Lakoff, Andrew. 2008. "From Population to Vital System: National Security and the Changing Object of Public Health." In *Biosecurity Interventions: Global Health and Security in Question*, edited by Andrew Lakoff and Stephen J. Collier, 33–60. New York: Columbia University Press.

Lakoff, Andrew. 2017. *Unprepared: Global Health in a Time of Emergency*. Berkeley: University of California Press.

The Lancet. 2015. "Global Health Security: The Wider Lessons from the West African Ebola Virus Disease Epidemic." *The Lancet* 385, no. 1: 1884–1901.

Larimer, Sarah. 2014a. "Police, Residents Clash in Liberian Slum under Ebola Quarantine." *Washington Post*, August 20, 2014. Retrieved from Factiva database.

Larimer, Sarah. 2014b. "Will the Ebola Virus Go Airborne? (And Is That Even the Right Question?)" *Washington Post*, September 16, 2014. Retrieved from Factiva database.

Layton, Lyndsey. 2014. "Kaci Hickox: 'Abundance of Politics' Led to Her N.J. Quarantine Over Ebola Fears." *Washington Post*, November 2, 2014. Retrieved from Factiva database.

Lazuta, Jennifer. 2014. "Ebola Toll Spreads Panic in West Africa." *USA Today*, April 3, 2014. Retrieved from Factiva database.

Leander, Anna and Ole Wæver. 2018. "Introduction." In *Assembling Exclusive Expertise: Knowledge, Ignorance and Conflict Resolution in the Global South*, edited by Anna Leander and Ole Wæver, 1–20. Abingdon, UK: Routledge.

Léonard, Sarah and Christian Kaunert. 2010. "Reconceptualizing the Audience in Securitization Theory." In *Securitization Theory: How Security Problems Emerge and Dissolve*, edited by Thierry Balzacq, 57–76. Abingdon, UK: Routledge.

Liu, Joanne. 2014. *MSF International President United Nations Special Briefing on Ebola*. Médecins Sans Frontières. https://www.msf.org/msf-international-president-united-nations-special-briefing-ebola.

Liptak, Kevin. 2014. "Obama Hits Road to Deal With Pair of Global Crises." *CNN*, September 15, 2014. Retrieved from Factiva database.

Lo, Catherine Yuk-Ping. 2015. *HIV/AIDS in China and India: Governing Health Security*. New York: Palgrave Macmillan.

Loewenson, Rene, Kirsten Accoe, Nitin Bajpai, Kent Buse, Thilagawathi Abi Deivanayaham, Leslie London, Claudio A Méndez, Tolib Mirzoev, Erica Nelson, Ateeb Ahmad Parray, Ari Probandari, Eric Sarriot, Moses Tetui, and André Janse van Rensburg. 2020. "Reclaiming Comprehensive Public Health." *BMJ Global Health* 5, no. 9: 1–5.

Lund Petersen, Karen. 2011. "Risk Analysis—a Field within Security Studies?" *European Journal of International Relations* 18, no. 4: 693–717.

Maclean, Sandra J. 2008. "Microbes, Mad Cows and Militaries: Exploring the Links Between Health and Security." *Security Dialogue* 39, no. 5: 475–494.

Marcos, Cristina. 2014. "House Republican to Introduce Ebola Travel Ban Legislation." *The Hill*, October 16, 2014. https://thehill.com/blogs/floor-action/house/220980-house-republican-to-introduce-bill-to-ban-west-africa-travel.

Marcotte, Amanda. 2014. "Calm Down about Ebola Already." *USA Today*, October 17, 2014. Retrieved from Factiva database.

Marcus, Ruth. 2014. "The Virus You Should Worry About." *Washington Post*, October 15, 2014. Retrieved from Factiva database.

Mastrangelo, Dominick. 2020. "Rand Paul Says Fauci Owes Parents and Students an Apology over Pandemic Measures." *The Hill*, November 30, 2014. https://thehill.com/homenews/527975-rand-paul-says-fauci-owes-parents-and-students-an-apology-over-pandemic-measures/.

Mbembe, Achille. 2019. *Necropolitics*. Translated by Steven Corcoran. Durham: Duke University Press.

McCoy, Terrence. 2014a. "Can Anything Stop West Africa's Outbreak of Ebola?" *Washington Post*, June 10, 2014. Retrieved from Factiva database.

McCoy, Terrence. 2014b. "This Is Now the Deadliest Ebola Outbreak on Record—and It's Getting Worse." *Washington Post*, June 27, 2014. Retrieved from Factiva database.

McCoy, Terrence. 2014c. "How Deforestation Shares the Blame for the Ebola Epidemic." *Washington Post*, July 11, 2014. Retrieved from Factiva database.

McCoy, Terrence. 2014d. "Two Infected Americans, a Dead Liberian Doctor, and the Worst-Ever Ebola Outbreak." *Washington Post*, August 1, 2014. Retrieved from Factiva database.

McCoy, Terrence. 2014e. "The Challenge of Stopping Ebola When It Keeps Killing Doctors." *Washington Post*, August 12, 2014. Retrieved from Factiva database.

McCoy, Terrence. 2014f. "Why the Escape of Numerous Ebola Patients in Liberia's Worst Slum Is So Terrifying." *Washington Post*, August 18, 2014. Retrieved from Factiva database.

McDonald, Matt. 2002. "Human Security and the Construction of Security." *Global Society* 16, no. 3: 277–295.

McDonald, Matt. 2003. "Environment and Security: Global Ecopolitics and Brazilian Deforestation." *Contemporary Security Policy* 24, no. 2: 69–94.

McDonald, Matt. 2008. "Securitization and the Construction of Security." *European Journal of International Relations* 14, no. 4: 563–587.

McDonald, Matt. 2012. "The Failed Securitization of Climate Change in Australia." *Australian Journal of Political Science* 47, no. 4: 579–592.

McInnes, Colin. 2005. "Health, Security, and the Risk Society." *Nuffield Trust*, November 15, 2005. https://www.nuffieldtrust.org.uk/resource/health-security-and-the-risk-society.

McInnes, Colin. 2014. "The Many Meanings of Health Security." In *Routledge Handbook of Global Health Security*, edited by Simon Rushton and Jeremy Youde, 7–17. Abingdon, UK: Routledge.

McInnes, Colin. 2016. "Crisis! What Crisis? Global Health and the 2014–15 West African Ebola Outbreak." *Third World Quarterly* 37, no. 3: 380–400.

McInnes, Colin and Kelley Lee. 2012. *Global Health and International Relations*. Cambridge: Polity.

McInnes, Colin and Anne Roemer-Mahler. 2017. "From Security to Risk: Reframing Global Health Threats." *International Affairs* 93, no. 6: 1313–1337.

McInnes, Colin and Simon Rushton. 2013. "HIV/AIDS and Securitization Theory." *European Journal of International Relations* 19, no. 1: 115–138.

McNeil, Donald G. Jr. 2014a. "Ebola, Killing Scores in Guinea, Threatens Nearby Nations." *New York Times*, March 25, 2014. Retrieved from Factiva database.

McNeil, Donald G. Jr. 2014b. "Using a Tactic Unseen in a Century, Countries Cordon Off Ebola-Racked Areas." *New York Times*, August 12, 2014. Retrieved from Factiva database.

Meet the Press (MTP). 2014a. Broadcast transcript. *NBC*, August 3, 2014. Retrieved from Factiva database.

MTP. 2014b. Broadcast transcript. *NBC*, September 7, 2014. Retrieved from Factiva database.

MTP. 2014c. Broadcast transcript. *NBC*, October 12, 2014. Retrieved from Factiva database.

MTP. 2014d. Broadcast transcript. *NBC*, November 2, 2014. Retrieved from Factiva database.

Metzgar, Emily. 2014. "Is U.S. 'Stuck on Stupid' with Ebola?" *USA Today*, October 22, 2014. Retrieved from Factiva database.

Milliken, Jennifer. 1999. "The Study of Discourse in International Relations: A Critique of Research and Methods." *European Journal of International Relations* 5, no. 2: 225–254.

Molnár, Anna, Lili Takács, and Éva Jakusné Harnos. 2020. "Securitization of the COVID-19 Pandemic by Metaphoric Discourse during the State of Emergency in Hungary." *International Journal of Sociology and Social Policy* 40, no. 9/10: 1167–1182.

Mui, Ylan Q. 2014. "Why Africa Will Remain an Economic Powerhouse despite the Ebola Virus." *Washington Post*, October 8, 2014. Retrieved from Factiva database.

Muller, Benjamin J. 2004. "(Dis)Qualified Bodies: Securitization, Citizenship and 'Identity Management.'" *Citizenship Studies* 8, no. 3: 279–294.

Muller, Benjamin J. 2008. "Securing the Political Imagination: Popular Culture, the Security Dispositif, and the Biometric State." *Security Dialogue* 39, no. 2–3: 199–220.

Murphy, Michael P. A. 2020. "COVID-19 and Emergency eLearning." *Contemporary Security Policy*, 41, no. 3: 492–505.

Musu, Constanza. 2020. "War Metaphors Used for COVID-19 Are Compelling but Also Dangerous." *The Conversation*, April 8, 2020. https://theconversation.com/war -metaphors-used-for-COVID-19-are-compelling-but-also-dangerous-135406.

MSNBC. 2014. Broadcast transcript. *MSNBC Vote!*, November 4, 2014. Retrieved from Factiva database.

Nakamura, David. 2014a. "Obama: Ebola is 'Growing Threat to Regional and Global Security.'" *Washington Post*, September 26, 2014. Retrieved from Factiva database.

Nakamura, David. 2014b. "Despite Some Concerns, Obama Administration Offers Support for House Spending Bill." *Washington Post*, December 11, 2014. Retrieved from Factiva database.

Neal, Andrew W. 2009. "Securitization and Risk at the EU Border: The Origins of FRONTEX." *Journal of Common Market Studies* 47, no. 2: 333–356.

Neal, Andrew W. 2010. *Exceptionalism and the Politics of Counter-Terrorism: Liberty, Security and the War on Terror*. London: Routledge.

Neal, Andrew W. 2019. *Security as Politics: Beyond the State of Exception*. Edinburgh: Edinburgh University Press.

New York City (NYC). 2014. "Mayor de Blasio, Governor Cuomo and New York City Health Officials Host Press Conference at Bellevue Hospital." Transcript. October 23, 2014. https://www1.nyc.gov/office-of-the-mayor/news/886-14/mayor-de-blasio -governor-cuomo-new-york-city-health-officials-host-press-conference-at.

New York Times Editorial Board (NYT). 2014a. "Obama's Africa Summit." *New York Times*, August 6, 2014. Retrieved from Factiva database.

NYT. 2014b. "Controlling the Ebola Epidemic." *New York Times*, August 11, 2014. Retrieved from Factiva database.

NYT. 2014c. "A Painfully Slow Ebola Response." *New York Times*, August 16, 2014. Retrieved from Factiva database.

NYT. 2014d. "India's Public Health Crisis." *New York Times*, October 18, 2014. Retrieved from Factiva database.

NYT. 2014e. "Negativity Wins the Senate." *New York Times*, November 5, 2014. Retrieved from Factiva database.

NYT. 2015. "Mission Not Yet Accomplished." *New York Times*, February 17, 2014. Retrieved from Factiva database.

Newsroom. 2014a. Broadcast transcript. *CNN*, April 15, 2014. Retrieved from Factiva database.

Newsroom. 2014b. Broadcast transcript. *CNN*, August 2, 2014. Retrieved from Factiva database.

Newsroom. 2014c. Broadcast transcript. *CNN*, August 3, 2014. Retrieved from Factiva database.

Newsroom. 2014d. Broadcast transcript. *CNN*, August 5, 2014. Retrieved from Factiva database.

Newsroom. 2014e. Broadcast transcript. *CNN*, August 6, 2014. Retrieved from Factiva database.

Newsroom. 2014f. Broadcast transcript. *CNN*, September 16, 2014. Retrieved from Factiva database.

Newsroom. 2014g. Broadcast transcript. *CNN*, September 17, 2014. Retrieved from Factiva database.

Newsroom. 2014h. Broadcast transcript. *CNN*, October 1, 2014. Retrieved from Factiva database.

Newsroom. 2014i. Broadcast transcript. *CNN*, October 23, 2014. Retrieved from Factiva database.

Newsroom. 2014j. Broadcast transcript. *CNN* October 26, 2014. Retrieved from Factiva database.

Newsroom. 2014k. Broadcast transcript. *CNN*, November 11, 2014. Retrieved from Factiva database.

Nightly News. 2014a. Broadcast transcript. *NBC*, April 14, 2014. Retrieved from Factiva database.

Nightly News. 2014b. Broadcast transcript. *NBC*, August 2, 2014. Retrieved from Factiva database.

Nightly News. 2014c. Broadcast transcript. *NBC*, September 16, 2014. Retrieved from Factiva database.

Noack, Rick. 2014. "Why Ebola Worries the Defense Department." *Washington Post*, August 6, 2014. Retrieved from Factiva database.

Nocera, Joe. 2014. "Failures of Competence." *New York Times*, October 18, 2014. Retrieved from Factiva database.

Nossiter, Adam. 2014a. "Ebola Reaches Guinean Capital, Stirring Fears." *New York Times*, April 2, 2014. Retrieved from Factiva database.

Nossiter, Adam. 2014b. "Ebola Rages in Guinea as Fear Keeps Help at Bay; Aid Workers Mistrusted by Villagers Are Meeting with Threats and Hostility." *New York Times*, July 26, 2014. Retrieved from Factiva database.

Nossiter, Adam. 2014c. "The Other Ebola Toll: African Economies." *New York Times*, September 6, 2014. Retrieved from Factiva database.

Nossiter, Adam. 2014d. "The Reality of Ebola, a World Away." *New York Times*, September 17, 2014. Retrieved from Factiva database.

Nossiter, Adam. 2014e. "Ebola: A Grave Site Report." *New York Times* (blog), September 23, 2014. Retrieved from Factiva database.

Nossiter, Adam. 2014f. "Ebola Epidemic Worsening, Sierra Leone Increases Quarantine Restrictions." *New York Times*, September 26, 2014. Retrieved from Factiva database.

Nossiter, Adam and Ben C. Solomon. 2014. "If They Survive in Ebola Ward, They Work On." *New York Times*, August 24, 2014. Retrieved from Factiva database.

Nunes, João. 2014a. "Questioning Health Security: Insecurity and Domination in World Politics." *Review of International Studies* 40, no. 5: 939–960.

Nunes, João. 2014b. *Security, Emancipation, and the Politics of Health*. Abingdon, UK: Routledge.

Nunes, João. 2016. "Ebola and the Production of Neglect in Global Health." *Third World Quarterly* 37, no 3: 542–556.

Nunes, João. 2017. "Doctors against Borders: Médecins Sans Frontières and Global Health Security." In *The Politics of Fear: Médecins Sans Frontières and the West African Ebola Epidemic*, edited by Michel Hofman and Sokhieng Au, 1–25. New York: Oxford University Press.

Nunes, João. 2020. "The COVID-19 Pandemic: Securitization, Neoliberal Crisis, and Global Vulnerabilization." *Cadernos de Saúde Pública* 36, no. 5: e00063120.

O'Connell, Stephen. 2014. "Washington Post Overly Alarmist on Liberia's 'Descent into Hell.'" *USAID* (blog), October 3, 2014. https://blog.usaid.gov/2014/10/washington-post-overly-alarmist-on-liberias-descent-into-hell/.

O'Manique, Colleen and Sandra J. MacLean. 2010. "Pathways Among Human Security, Gender, and HIV/AIDS in Sub-Saharan Africa." *Canadian Journal of African Studies* 44, no. 3: 457–478.

The O'Reilly Factor (TOF). 2014a. Broadcast transcript. *Fox News*, October 1, 2014. Retrieved from Factiva database.

TOF. 2014b. Broadcast transcript. *Fox News*, October 3, 2014. Retrieved from Factiva database.

TOF. 2014c. Broadcast transcript. *Fox News*, October 13, 2014. Retrieved from Factiva database.

TOF. 2014d. Broadcast transcript. *Fox News*, October 17, 2014. Retrieved from Factiva database.

TOF. 2014e. Broadcast transcript. *Fox News*, October 27, 2014. Retrieved from Factiva database.

Obama, Barack. 2014a. "Remarks by the President at Press Conference After U.S.-Africa Leaders Summit." Transcript. Obama White House Archives (website). August 6, 2014. https://obamawhitehouse.archives.gov/the-press-office/2014/08/06/remarks-president-press-conference-after-us-africa-leaders-summit.

Obama, Barack. 2014b. "Remarks by the President on the Ebola Outbreak." Transcript. Obama White House Archives (website). September 16, 2014. https://obamawhitehouse.archives.gov/the-press-office/2014/09/16/remarks-president-ebola-outbreak.

Obama, Barack. 2014c. "Remarks by the President at MacDill Air Force Base." Transcript. Obama White House Archives (website). September 17, 2014. https://obamawhitehouse.archives.gov/the-press-office/2014/09/17/remarks-president-macdill-air-force-base.

Obama, Barack. 2014d. "Remarks by President Obama in Address to the United Nations General Assembly." Transcript. Obama White House Archives (website). September 24, 2014. https://obamawhitehouse.archives.gov/the-press-office/2014/09/24/remarks-president-obama-address-united-nations-general-assembly.

Obama, Barack. 2014e. "Remarks by President Obama at U.N. Meeting on Ebola." Transcript. Obama White House Archives (website). September 25, 2014. https://obamawhitehouse.archives.gov/the-press-office/2014/09/25/remarks-president-obama-un-meeting-ebola.

Obama, Barack. 2014f. "Remarks by the President at Global Health Security Agenda Summit." Transcript. Obama White House Archives (website). September 26, 2014. https://obamawhitehouse.archives.gov/the-press-office/2014/09/26/remarks-president-global-health-security-agenda-summit.

Obama, Barack. 2014g. "Remarks by the President After Meeting on Ebola." Transcript. Obama White House Archives (website). October 6, 2014. https://obamawhitehouse.archives.gov/the-press-office/2014/10/06/remarks-president-after-meeting-ebola.

Obama, Barack. 2014h. "Weekly Address: What You Need to Know About Ebola." Transcript. Obama White House Archives (website). October 18, 2014. https://obamawhitehouse.archives.gov/the-press-office/2014/10/18/weekly-address-what-you-need-know-about-ebola.

Obama, Barack. 2014i. "Remarks by the President on Ebola." Transcript. Obama White House Archives (website). October 28, 2014. https://obamawhitehouse.archives.gov/the-press-office/2014/10/28/remarks-president-ebola.

Obama, Barack. 2014j. "Letter from the President—Emergency Appropriations Request for Ebola for Fiscal Year 2015." Letter. Obama White House Archives (website). November 5, 2014. https://obamawhitehouse.archives.gov/the-press-office /2014/11/05/letter-president-emergency-appropriations-request-ebola-fiscal-year-2015.

Obama, Barack. 2014k. "Remarks by the President on Research for Potential Ebola Vaccines." Transcript. Obama White House Archives (website). December 2, 2014. https://obamawhitehouse.archives.gov/the-press-office/2014/12/02/remarks-presi dent-research-potential-ebola-vaccines.

Obama, Barack. 2015. "Remarks by the President on America's Leadership in the Ebola Fight." Transcript. Obama White House Archives (website). February 11, 2015. https://obamawhitehouse.archives.gov/the-press-office/2015/02/11/remarks-presi dent-americas-leadership-ebola-fight.

Ogata, Sadako and Amartya Sen. 2003. *Human Security Now*. New York: Commission on Human Security. https://digitallibrary.un.org/record/503749?ln=en

Ohlheiser, Abby. 2014. "It's Highly Unlikely That You'll Become Infected with Ebola. So What Are You So Afraid Of?" *Washington Post*, October 6, 2014. Retrieved from Factiva database.

Onishi, Norimitsu. 2014a. "Clashes Erupt as Liberia Sets a Quarantine." *New York Times*, August 21, 2014. Retrieved from Factiva database.

Onishi, Norimitsu. 2014b. "Back to the Slums of His Youth, to Defuse the Ebola Time Bomb." *New York Times*, September 14, 2014. Retrieved from Factiva database.

Onishi, Norimitsu and Jad Mouawad. 2014. "Ebola Patient's Journey Shows How Global Travel Is Open to Spread of Disease." *New York Times*, October 3, 2014. Retrieved from Factiva database.

Ostergard, Robert L. 2002. "Politics in the Hot Zone: Aids and National Security in Africa." *Third World Quarterly* 23, no. 2: 333–350.

Osterholm, Michael T. 2007. "Unprepared For a Pandemic." *Foreign Affairs* 86, no. 2: 47–57.

Osterholm, Michael T. 2014a. "What We Need to Fight Ebola." *Washington Post*, August 1, 2014. Retrieved from Factiva database.

Osterholm, Michael T. 2014b. "What We're Afraid to Say about Ebola." *New York Times*, September 12, 2014. Retrieved from Factiva database.

Owen, Taylor. 2004. "Human Security—Conflict, Critique and Consensus: Collo-quium Remarks and a Proposal for a Threshold-Based Definition." *Security Dialogue* 35, no. 3: 373–387.

Paris, Roland. 2001. "Human Security: Paradigm Shift or Hot Air?" *International Security* 26, no 2: 87–102.

Parker, Kathleen. 2014. "Political Pendulum Swings Right." *Washington Post*, November 2, 2014. Retrieved from Factiva database.

Parker, Ashley and Jonathan Weisman. 2014. "Big Concessions Mark U.S. Deal on Spending." *New York Times*, December 11, 2014. Retrieved from Factiva database.

Parker, Melissa, Hayley MacGregor, and Grace Akello. 2020. "COVID-19, Public Authority and Enforcement." *Medical Anthropology*, 39, no. 8: 666–670.

Paye-Layleh, Jonathon. 2014. "In Liberia, Ebola Fears Rising." *Washington Post*, August 18, 2014. Retrieved from Factiva database.

Perez-Pena, Richard. 2014. "Alarmed by Ebola, Public Isn't Calmed by 'Experts Say.'" *New York Times*, November 1, 2014. Retrieved from Factiva database.

Petersen, Susan. 2002. "Epidemic Disease and National Security." *Security Studies* 12, no. 2: 43–81.

Petrow, Steven. 2014. "Why 'Fearbola' Reminds Me of the Early Aids Panic." *Washington Post*, October 15, 2014. Retrieved from Factiva database.

Piot, Peter. 2014. "Ebola's Perfect Storm." *Science* 345, no. 6202: 1221.

Politics Nation (PN). 2014a. Broadcast transcript. *MSNBC*, October 9, 2014. Retrieved from Factiva database.

PN. 2014b. Broadcast transcript. *MSNBC*, October 28, 2014. Retrieved from Factiva database.

Pollack, Andrew. 2014a. "In Ebola Outbreak, Who Should Get Experimental Drug?" *New York Times*, August 9, 2014. Retrieved from Factiva database.

Pollack, Andrew. 2014b. "Stabbing with Syringe in Nigeria Raises Concerns of Ebola as Weapon." *New York Times*, September 11, 2014. Retrieved from Factiva database.

Price-Smith, Andrew T. 2009. *Contagion and Chaos: Disease, Ecology, and National Security in the Era of Globalization*. Cambridge, MA: MIT Press.

Quammen, David. 2014. "Ebola Virus: A Grim, African Reality." *New York Times*, April 10, 2014. Retrieved from Factiva database.

The Rachel Maddow Show (TRMS). 2014a. Broadcast transcript. *MSNBC*, October 1, 2014. Retrieved from Factiva database.

TRMS. 2014b. Broadcast transcript. *MSNBC*, October 2, 2014. Retrieved from Factiva database.

TRMS. 2014c. Broadcast transcript. *MSNBC*, October 30, 2014. Retrieved from Factiva database.

Reliable Sources. 2014a. Broadcast transcript. *CNN*, October 5, 2014. Retrieved from Factiva database.

Reliable Sources. 2014b. Broadcast transcript. *CNN*, November 2, 2014. Retrieved from Factiva database.

Rice, Susan. E. 2014. "Opening Remarks by National Security Advisor Susan E. Rice at the Global Health Security Agenda Conference." Transcript. Obama White House Archives (website). September 26, 2014. https://obamawhitehouse.archives.gov/the -press-office/2014/09/26/opening-remarks-national-security-advisor-susan-e-rice -global-health-sec.

Robbins, Mel. 2014. "'Fear-Bola' Hits Epidemic Proportions." *CNN*, October 15, 2014. http://edition.cnn.com/2014/10/15/opinion/robbins-ebola-fear/.

Roberts, Stephen L. 2019. "Big Data, Algorithmic Governmentality and the Regulation of Pandemic Risk." *European Journal of Risk Regulation* 10, no. 1: 94–115.

Roberts, Stephen L. and Stefan Elbe. 2016. "Catching the Flu: Syndromic Surveillance, Algorithmic Governmentality and Global Health Security." *Security Dialogue* 48, no. 1: 46–62.

Roe, Paul. 2008. "Actor, Audience(s) and Emergency Measures: Securitization and the UK's Decision to Invade Iraq." *Security Dialogue* 39, no. 6: 615–635.

Roemer-Mahler, Anne and Stefan Elbe. 2016. "The Race for Ebola Drugs: Pharmaceuticals, Security and Global Health Governance." *Third World Quarterly* 37, no. 3: 487–506.

Root Wolpe, Paul. 2014. "Heroic Americans with Ebola Should Be Welcomed Home." *CNN*, August 5, 2014. Retrieved from Factiva database.

Rosenthal, Andrew. 2014. "No Comment Necessary: Blaming the Ebola Victim." *New York Times* (blog), August 7, 2014. Retrieved from Factiva database.

Rothschild, Emma. 1995. "What is Security?" *Daedalus* 124, no. 3: 53–98.

Rubin, Jennifer. 2014a. "A Presidential Candidate in the Age of Anxiety." *Washington Post*, October 15, 2014. Retrieved from Factiva database.

Rubin, Jennifer. 2014b. "Libertarian Message Wasn't the Ticket to the GOP Wave." *Washington Post*, November 5, 2014. Retrieved from Factiva database.

Rushe, Dominic. 2014. "Isolated Nurse Slams Chris Christie's Ebola Quarantine Policy." *Guardian*, October 27, 2014. https://www.theguardian.com/world/2014/oct /26/ebola-christie-quarantine-west-africa-monitor-symptoms-airport.

Rushton, Simon. 2011. "Global Health Security: Security for Whom? Security from What?" *Political Studies* 59, no. 4: 779–796.

Rushton, Simon. 2019. *Security and Public Health: Pandemics and Politics in the Contemporary World*. Cambridge: Polity.

Rushton, Simon. 2022. "Can We Rely on the Security Council during Health Emergencies?" *Australian Journal of International Affairs* 76, no. 1: 35–39.

Russell, Cristine. 2016. "Risk Watch: Media Coverage of Ebola in the Digital Communication Era." In *Ebola's Message*, edited by Nicholas G. Evans, Tara C. Smith, and Maimuna S. Majumder, 141–155. Cambridge, MA: MIT Press.

Rutledge, Paul E. 2020. "Trump, COVID-19, and the War on Expertise." *American Review of Public Administration* 50, no. 6–7: 505–511.

Sack, Kevin, Jack Healy, and Frances Robles. 2014. "Life in Quarantine for Ebola Exposure: 21 Days of Fear and Loathing." *New York Times*, October 19, 2014. Retrieved from Factiva database.

Salter, Mark. 2008a. "Imagining Numbers: Risk, Quantification, and Aviation Security." *Security Dialogue* 39, no. 2–3: 243–266.

Salter, Mark. 2008b. "Securitization and Desecuritization: A Dramaturgical Analysis of the Canadian Air Transport Security Authority." *Journal of International Relations and Development* 11, no. 4: 321–349.

Sanburn, Josh. 2014. "Ebola Brings Another Fear: Xenophobia." *Time*, October 29, 2014. https://time.com/3544130/ebola-panic-xenophobia/.

Sandset, Tony. 2021. "The Necropolitics of COVID-19: Race, Class, and Slow Death in an Ongoing Pandemic." *Global Public Health* 16, no. 8–9: 1411–1423.

Sanjay Gupta MD (SGMD). 2014. Broadcast transcript. August 9, 2014. Retrieved from Factiva database.

Santora, Marc. 2014a. "Doctor in New York City Is Sick with Ebola." *New York Times*, October 24, 2014. Retrieved from Factiva database.

Santora, Marc. 2014b. "First Patient Quarantined Under Strict New Policy Tests Negative for Ebola." *New York Times*, October 25, 2014. Retrieved from Factiva database.

Sargent, Greg. 2014. "Morning Plum: Jeb Bush Again Challenges Republicans on Immigration." *Washington Post*, December 2, 2014. Retrieved from Factiva database.

Schmemann, Serge. 2014a. "A Peaceful Decision in Scotland, but Misery Elsewhere." *New York Times*, September 21, 2014. Retrieved from Factiva database.

Schmemann, Serge. 2014b. "Ebola Alarm, Rebellion in Europe and Turkey's Puzzling Attack." *New York Times*, October 19, 2014. Retrieved from Factiva database.

Schmitt, Carl. (1922) 2005. *Political Theology: Four Chapters on the Concept of Sovereignty*, translated by G. Schwab. Chicago: Chicago University Press.

Schmitt, Carl. (1932) 2010. *The Concept of the Political*, translated by G. Schwab. Chicago: University of Chicago Press.

Seay, Laura. 2014. "Ebola, Research Ethics, and the ZMapp Serum." *Washington Post*, August 6, 2014. Retrieved from Factiva database.

Seay, Laura and Kim Yi Dionne. 2014. "The Long and Ugly Tradition of Treating Africa as a Dirty, Diseased Place." *Washington Post*, August 25, 2014. Retrieved from Factiva database.

Sekalala, Sharifah, Caitlin R. Williams, and Benjamin Mason Meier. 2022. "Global Health Governance through the Un Security Council: Health Security vs. Human Rights?" *Australian Journal of International Affairs* 76, no. 1: 27–34.

Sengupta, Somini. 2014. "Ebola Presents Challenge, and an Opportunity, for UN Leader." *New York Times*, September 19, 2014. Retrieved from Factiva database.

Sengupta, Somini, Rick Gladstone, and Sheri Fink. 2014. "UN Leader Plans Effort to Aid Ebola Struggle." *New York Times*, September 18, 2014. Retrieved from Factiva database.

Shepard Smith Reporting (SSR). 2014. Broadcast transcript. *Fox News*, October 15, 2014. Retrieved from Factiva database.

Shear, Michael D. and Mark Landler. 2014. "Amid Assurances on Ebola, Obama Is Said to Seethe." *New York Times*, October 17, 2014. Retrieved from Factiva database.

Shepherd, Laura. 2021. *Narrating the Women, Peace, and Security Agenda*. New York: Oxford.

Shklar, Judith. 1998. "The Liberalism of Fear." In *Political Thought and Political Thinkers*, edited by Stanley Hoffman, 3–20. Chicago: University of Chicago Press.

Siegel, Marc. 2014. "Ebola Doctors Sacrifice All to Bring Hope; Like Aids Outbreak, They Work Front Lines." *USA Today*, August 1, 2014. Retrieved from Factiva database.

The Situation Room (TSR). 2014a. Broadcast transcript. *CNN*, August 7, 2014. Retrieved from Factiva database.

TSR. 2014b. Broadcast transcript. *CNN*, September 16, 2014. Retrieved from Factiva database.

TSR. 2014c. Broadcast transcript. *CNN*, September 30, 2014. Retrieved from Factiva database.

TSR. 2014d. Broadcast transcript. *CNN*, October 2, 2014. Retrieved from Factiva database.

TSR. 2014e. Broadcast transcript. *CNN*, October 24, 2014. Retrieved from Factiva database.

TSR. 2014f. Broadcast transcript. *CNN*, November 14, 2014. Retrieved from Factiva database.

Sjöstedt, Roxanna. 2008. "Exploring the Construction of Threats: The Securitization of HIV/AIDS in Russia." *Security Dialogue* 39, no. 1: 7–29.

Slaven, Mike. 2021. "Populism and Securitization: The Corrosion of Elite Security Authority in a US-Mexico Border State." *Journal of Global Security Studies* 6, no. 4: 1–18.

Smith, Stephanie. "The Roots of Our Ebola Fears." *CNN*, August 6, 2014. Retrieved from Factiva database.

Somin, Ilya. 2014. "Ebola, Political Ignorance, and the Undead." *Washington Post*, November 1, 2014. Retrieved from Factiva database.

Sondermann, Elena, and Cornelia Ulbert. 2020. "The Threat of Thinking in Threats: Reframing Global Health during and after COVID-19." *Zeitschrift für Friedens- und Konfliktforschung*, 9, no. 2: 309–320.

Song, Weiqing. 2015. "Securitization of the 'China Threat' Discourse: A Poststructuralist Account." *China Review* 15, no. 1: 145–169.

Special Report with Bret Baier (SRBB). 2014a. Broadcast transcript. *Fox News*, August 1, 2014. Retrieved from Factiva database.

SRBB. 2014b. Broadcast transcript. *Fox News*, August 5, 2014. Retrieved from Factiva database.

SRBB. 2014c. Broadcast transcript. *Fox News*, August 6, 2014. Retrieved from Factiva database.

SRBB. 2014d. Broadcast transcript. *Fox News*, September 15, 2014. Retrieved from Factiva database.

SRBB. 2014e. Broadcast transcript. *Fox News*, September 16, 2014. Retrieved from Factiva database.

SRBB. 2014f. Broadcast transcript. *Fox News*, October 13, 2014. Retrieved from Factiva database.

SRBB. 2014g. Broadcast transcript. *Fox News*, October 27, 2014. Retrieved from Factiva database.

State of the Union (SOTU). 2014a. Broadcast transcript. *CNN*, September 28, 2014. Retrieved from Factiva database.

SOTU. 2014b. Broadcast transcript. *CNN*, October 19, 2014. Retrieved from Factiva database.

SOTU. 2014c. Broadcast transcript. *CNN*, October 26, 2014. Retrieved from Factiva database.

Steinhauer, Jennifer. 2014. "Fear of Ebola Closes Schools and Shapes Politics." *New York Times*, October 20, 2014. Retrieved from Factiva database.

Stop Ebola Act. 2014. H.R. 5688. 113th Congress. Retrieved from https://www.con gress.gov/bill/113th-congress/house-bill/5688.

Stott, Clifford, Owen West, and Mark Harrison. 2020. "A Turning Point, Securitization, and Policing in the Context of COVID-19: Building a New Social Contract Between State and Nation?" *Policing: A Journal of Policy and Practice* 14, no. 3: 574–578.

Strain, Michael R. 2014. "Americans Have Already Forgotten That This Is a Great Nation." *Washington Post*, September 10, 2014. Retrieved from Factiva database.

Stritzel, Holger. 2007. "Towards a Theory of Securitization: Copenhagen and Beyond." *European Journal of International Relations* 13, no. 3: 357–383.

Stritzel, Holger. 2012. "Securitization, Power, Intertextuality: Discourse Theory and the Translations of Organized Crime." *Security Dialogue* 43, no. 6: 549–567.

Stritzel, Holger. 2014. *Security as Translation: Securitization Theory and the Localization of Threat*. Basingstroke, Hampshire: Palgrave Macmillan.

Sullivan, Gail. 2014a. "Gov. Christie's Ebola Quarantine Messed with the 'Wrong Redhead.'" *Washington Post*, October 27, 2014. Retrieved from Factiva database.

Sullivan, Gail. 2014b. "Report: After fight with Chris Christie, nurse Kaci Hickox will defy Ebola quarantine in Maine." *Washington Post*, October 29, 2014. Retrieved from Factiva database.

Sullivan, Sean. 2014. "Chris Christie Took a Hard Line on Ebola. It Could Come Back to Bite Him." *Washington Post*, October 27, 2014. Retrieved from Factiva database.

Sun, Lena H. and Juliet Eilperin. 2014. "U.S. Military to Help Fight Ebola in Africa." *Washington Post*, September 8, 2014. Retrieved from Factiva database.

Sun, Lena H., Brady Dennis, Lenny Bernstein, and Joel Achenbach. 2014. "Out of Control: How the World's Health Organizations Failed to Stop the Ebola Disaster." *Washington Post*, October 5, 2014. Retrieved from Factiva database.

Tjalve, Vibeke Schou. 2011. "Designing (De)Security: European Exceptionalism, Atlantic Republicanism and the 'Public Sphere.'" *Security Dialogue* 42, no. 4–5: 441–452.

Today. 2014a. Broadcast transcript. *NBC*, August 1, 2014. Retrieved from Factiva database.

Today. 2014b. Broadcast transcript. *NBC*, August 5, 2014. Retrieved from Factiva database.

Today. 2014c. Broadcast transcript. *NBC*, October 1, 2014. Retrieved from Factiva database.

Topaz, Jonathan. 2014. "Jindal: Ban Travel from Ebola Nations." *Politico*, October 3, 2014. https://www.politico.com/story/2014/10/ebola-travel-bobby-jindal-comments -111592.

Trombetta, Maria Julia. 2008. "Environmental Security and Climate Change: Analysing the Discourse." *Cambridge Review of International Affairs* 21, no. 4: 585–602.

Trump, Donald (@realDonaldTrump). 2014. "The U.S. cannot allow EBOLA infected people back. People that go to far away places to help out are great-but must suffer the consequences!" Twitter, August 2, 2014. 11:22 a.m. Accessed via the Trump Twitter Archive.

USA Today. 2014a. "Fear Spreads Faster than Ebola." October 15, 2014. Retrieved from Factiva database.

USA Today. 2014b. "Governors' Hasty Quarantine Adds to Ebola Problems." October 28, 2014. Retrieved from Factiva database.

van Kolfschooten, Hannah, and Anniek de Ruijter. 2020. "COVID-19 and Privacy in the European Union: A Legal Perspective on Contact Tracing." *Contemporary Security Policy* 41, no. 3: 478–491.

van Rythoven, Eric. 2015. "Learning to Feel, Learning to Fear? Emotions, Imaginaries, and Limits in the Politics of Securitization." *Security Dialogue* 46, no. 5: 458–475.

van Rythoven, Eric (2020) "What's Wrong with the War Metaphor." *Duck of Minerva*, April 5, 2020. https://duckofminerva.com/2020/04/whats-wrong-with-the -war-metaphor.html.

Vankovska, Biljana. 2020. "Dealing With COVID-19 in the European Periphery: Between Securitization and 'Gaslighting.'" *Journal of Global Faultlines*, 7, no. 1: 71–88.

Vaughn, Jocelyn. 2009. "The Unlikely Securitizer: Humanitarian Organizations and the Securitization of Indistinctiveness." *Security Dialogue* 40, no. 3: 263–285.

Ventura, Deisy De Freitas Lima. 2016. "From Ebola to Zika: International Emergencies and the Securitization of Global Health." *Cadernos de Saúde Pública* 32, no. 4: 1–4.

Voss, Maike, Isabell Kump, and Paul Bochtler. 2022. "Unpacking the Framing of Health in the United Nations Security Council." *Australian Journal of International Affairs* 76, no. 1: 4–10.

Vultee, Fred. 2010. "Securitization as a Media Frame: What Happens When the Media 'Speak Security.'" In *Securitization Theory: How Security Problems Emerge and Dissolve*, edited by Thierry Balzacq, 77–93. Abingdon, UK: Routledge.

Vuori, Juha A. 2008. "Illocutionary Logic and Strands of Securitization: Applying the Theory of Securitization to the Study of Non-Democratic Political Orders." *European Journal of International Relations* 14, no. 1: 65–99.

Wæver, Ole. 1995. "Securitization and Desecuritization." In *On Security*, edited by Ronnie D. Lipschutz. New York: Columbia University Press.

Wæver, Ole. 1999. "Securitizing Sectors? Reply to Eriksson." *Cooperation and Conflict* 34, no. 3: 334–340.

Wæver, Ole. 2011. "Politics, Security, Theory." *Security Dialogue* 42, no. 4–5: 465–480.

Wæver, Ole. 2015. "The Theory Act: Responsibility and Exactitude as Seen from Securitization." *International Relations* 29, no. 1: 121–128.

Wald, Priscilla. 2008. *Contagious: Cultures, Carriers, and the Outbreak Narrative.* Durham: Duke University Press.

Washington Post Editorial Board (WP). 2014a. "The Real Ebola Danger." August 6, 2014. Retrieved from Factiva database.

WP. 2014b. "Africa Summit Marks a Tectonic Shift That Should Be Bolstered." August 8, 2014. Retrieved from Factiva database.

WP. 2014c. "Combating Ebola." September 17, 2014. Retrieved from Factiva database.

WP. 2014d. "An Ebola Quarantine Is a Bad Idea." October 27, 2014. Retrieved from Factiva database.

WP. 2014e. "With Ebola, Exercise the Most Caution Possible." October 31, 2014. Retrieved from Factiva database.

WP. 2014f. "The Good and the Bad in Congress's Gargantuan Spending Bill." December 11, 2014. Retrieved from Factiva database.

Watson, Traci. 2014. "Ebola Fighters Charge Ahead to Tackle Crisis; Battling Virus Takes Physical, Emotional Toll on Volunteers Who Delve into Hot Zone." *USA Today*, September 26, 2014. Retrieved from Factiva database.

Watterson, Christopher and Adam Kamradt-Scott. 2016. "Fighting Flu: Securitization and the Military Role in Combating Influenza." *Armed Forces and Society* 42, no. 1: 145–168.

Weir, Lorna. 2014. "Inventing Global Health Security, 1994–2005." In *Routledge Handbook of Global Health Security*, edited by Simon Rushton and Jeremy Youde, 18–31. Abingdon, UK: Routledge.

Weir, Lorna and Eric Mykhalovskiy. 2010. *Global Public Health Vigilance: Creating a World on Alert.* New York: Routledge.

Weldes, Jutta. 1996. "Constructing National Interests." *European Journal of International Relations* 2, no. 3: 275–318.

Wemple, Erik. 2014. "Conspiracy Theory-Driven Fox News Doc Recently Scored Contract Renewal." *Washington Post*, October 17, 2014. Retrieved from Factiva database.

Wenham, Clare. 2016. "Ebola Respons-Ibility: Moving from Shared to Multiple Responsibilities." *Third World Quarterly* 37, no. 3: 426–451.

Wenham, Clare. 2019. "The Oversecuritization of Global Health: Changing the Terms of Debate." *International Affairs* 95, no. 5: 1093–1110.

Wenham, Clare. 2021. *Feminist Global Health Security*. New York: Oxford University Press.

Wenham, Clare and Deborah BL. Farias. 2019. "Securitizing Zika: The Case of Brazil." *Security Dialogue* 50, no. 5: 398–415.

Wickham, DeWayne. 2014a. "Obama Critics Off-Base over Ebola Travel Ban." *USA Today*, October 21, 2014. Retrieved from Factiva database.

Wickham, DeWayne. 2014b. "Why Not Quarantine for Common Influenza?" *USA Today*, November 11, 2014. Retrieved from Factiva database.

Wilhelmsen, Julie. 2017. "How Does War Become a Legitimate Undertaking? Re-Engaging the Post-structuralist Foundation of Securitization Theory." *Cooperation and Conflict* 52, no. 2: 166–183.

Williams, Michael C. 1998. "Identity and the Politics of Security." *European Journal of International Relations* 4, no. 2: 204–225.

Williams, Michael C. 2003. "Words, Images, Enemies: Securitization and International Politics." *International Studies Quarterly* 47, no. 4: 511–531.

Williams, Michael C. 2010. "The Continuing Evolution of Securitization Theory." In *Securitization Theory: How Security Problems Emerge and Dissolve*, edited by Thierry Balzacq, 212–222. Milton Park: Routledge.

Williams, Michael C. 2011. "Securitization and the Liberalism of Fear." *Security Dialogue* 42, no. 4–5: 453–463.

Williams, Michael C. 2015. "Securitization as Political Theory: The Politics of the Extraordinary." *International Relations* 29, no. 1: 114–120.

Wilson, Jacque. 2014. "Ebola Outbreak Could Have 'Catastrophic' Consequences." *CNN*, August 1, 2014. Retrieved from Factiva database.

Witte, Griff and Anna Fifield. 2014. "US Election Results Resonate Globally, with Fears of a Deepening Leadership Void." *Washington Post*, November 6, 2014. Retrieved from Factiva database.

Wishnick, Elizabeth. 2010. "Dilemmas of Securitization and Health Risk Management in the People's Republic of China: The Cases of SARS and Avian Influenza." *Health Policy and Planning* 25, no. 6: 454–466.

White House. 2014a. "Press Briefing by Press Secretary Josh Earnest." Transcript. Obama White House Archives (website). August 5, 2014. https://obamawhitehouse .archives.gov/the-press-office/2014/08/05/press-briefing-press-secretary-josh-earnest -8514

White House. 2014b. "Press Briefing by Press Secretary Josh Earnest." Transcript. Obama White House Archives (website). September 15, 2014. https://obamawhite house.archives.gov/the-press-office/2014/09/16/press-gaggle-press-secretary-josh -earnest-en-route-atlanta-georgia-91614.

White House. 2014c. "Daily Briefing by the Press Secretary." Transcript. Obama White House Archives (website). October 8, 2014. https://obamawhitehouse.archives.gov /the-press-office/2014/10/08/daily-briefing-press-secretary.

White House. 2014d. "Press Briefing by Press Secretary Josh Earnest." Transcript. Obama White House Archives (website). October 17, 2014. https://obamawhite house.archives.gov/the-press-office/2014/10/17/press-briefing-press-secretary-josh-earnest -101714.

White House. 2014e. "Press Gaggle by Press Secretary Josh Earnest en route Portland, ME." Transcript. Obama White House Archives (website). October 30, 2014. https:// obamawhitehouse.archives.gov/the-press-office/2014/10/30/press-gaggle-press -secretary-josh-earnest-en-route-portland-me-10302014.

White House. 2015. "FACT SHEET: Progress in Our Ebola Response at Home and Abroad." Obama White House Archives (website). February 11, 2014. https:// obamawhitehouse.archives.gov/the-press-office/2015/02/11/fact-sheet-progress-our -ebola-response-home-and-abroad.

World Health Organization (WHO). 2005. *International Health Regulations*. 3rd ed. Geneva: WHO Press.

WHO. 2014. *Ethical Considerations for Use of Unregistered Interventions for Ebola Viral Disease: Report of an Advisory Panel to WHO*. Geneva: Switzerland.

Yanzhong Huang. 2014. "The Downside of Securitizing the Ebola Virus." *Council on Foreign Relations Expert Brief*, November 25, 2014. https://www.cfr.org/expert-brief /downside-securitizing-ebola-virus.

Yong, Ed. 2020. "How the Pandemic Defeated America." *Atlantic*, September 15, 2014. https://www.theatlantic.com/magazine/archive/2020/09/coronavirus-american -failure/614191/.

Youde, Jeremy. 2010. *Biopolitical Surveillance and Public Health in International Politics*. New York: Palgrave Macmillan.

Youde, Jeremy. 2016. "High Politics, Low Politics, and Global Health." *Journal of Global Security Studies* 1, no. 2: 157–170.

Youde, Jeremy. 2018a. *Global Health Governance in International Society*. Oxford: Oxford University Press.

Youde, Jeremy. 2018b. "The Securitization of Health in the Trump Era." *Australian Journal of International Affairs* 72, no. 6: 535–550.

Youde, Jeremy and Simon Rushton. 2014. "Introduction." In *Routledge Handbook of Global Health Security*, edited by Simon Rushton and Jeremy Youde, 1–3. Abingdon, UK: Routledge.

Your World with Neil Cavuto (YWNC). 2014a. Broadcast transcript. *Fox News*, August 5, 2014. Retrieved from Factiva database.

YWNC. 2014b. Broadcast transcript. *Fox News*, October 1, 2014. Retrieved from Factiva database.

YWNC. 2014c. Broadcast transcript. *Fox News*, October 8, 2014. Retrieved from Factiva database.

YWNC. 2014d. Broadcast transcript. *Fox News*, October 10, 2014. Retrieved from Factiva database.

Index

Actors beyond elites, 46–48

Agency, 43, 55

Airport screenings, enhanced, 9, 17, 71, 115–116

Albright, Madeleine, 73

Alcabes, Phillip, 172

Alexander, Lamar, 70

America Under Threat (AUT) discourse
  audience and, 140
  authority and, 142
  contestation and, 159
  as dominant, 16, 17–18, 164–165
  Duncan and, 113
  evolution of, 106–107
  exceptionalism and, 155, 157–158
  Fearbola counterdiscourse and, 91, 92, 95, 118–119
  first appearance of, 103
  Hickox and, 124–125
  HWA discourse and, 104–105
  main examination of, 74–84
  midterm elections and, 125, 126, 128
  mutation and, 68
  Obama and, 111–112, 127, 131
  outbreak narrative and, 152
  PGC discourse and, 116, 129–130
  quarantines and, 121, 122
  racialization and, 171–172
  rise of, 29
  risk and, 144–145, 146
  Self/Other relationship and, 137–139

"success" and, 120

West African Fragility representation and, 97

Aradau, Claudia, 50, 51, 144, 156, 167

Atlas, Scott, 176

Attiah, Karen, 128

Audience
  contestation and, 135, 139–144
  Copenhagen School on, 38–39, 59
  Fearbola counterdiscourse and, 91–92
  main examination of, 41–44
  as performative, 43
  PGC discourse and, 72–73
  representations of, 101
  securitization theory and, 21, 22
  securitizing actors and, 47–48

Audience acceptance, 35–36, 38

Authority, 51, 71–72, 75–76, 101, 115, 135, 139–144

Authorization, 28, 44, 47, 56, 141

Balzacq, Thierry, 20, 23, 32, 39, 40, 41, 45, 151

Ban Ki-Moon, 130

Basic discourses, 61–62

Benton, Adia, 94

Berents, Helen, 87

Blitzer, Wolf, 114

Border security, 45. See also Immigration

Bourdieu, Pierre, 32

Brantly, Kent, 8, 73, 102–108, 111, 121,
    133, 142, 148
Brooks, David, 126
Brown, Scott, 125
Bubandt, Nils, 151
Burnett, Erin, 105, 121
Butler, Judith, 43, 55
Buzan, Barry, 19

Campbell, David, 22
Caremel, Jean-François, 38
Catastrophe, 51
Catastrophic damage, 63, 69
CDC
    Aeromedical Biological Containment
        System, 8
    airport screenings and, 9
    authority and, 117–118
    Obama and, 108, 109, 132, 154
    outbreak timeline and, 8
    speculation and, 106–107
    timing of response and, 147–149
Change, 22, 24, 32, 42, 45–46, 53–54,
    59, 92, 100, 170
Christie, Chris, 2, 9, 75, 82, 121–124,
    142, 174
Ciută, Felix, 34, 36, 151
Claim-making, field of, 44–45
Clinical holds, 83
Cohen, Elizabeth, 129
Coming Anarchy, The (Kaplan), 177
Constructed meaning, 48
Containment, 149
Content analysis, 56
Contestation, 38, 43–46, 53–54, 100, 107,
    123, 132, 135, 139–144, 159, 167
Context, role of, 38–39, 44–46, 48, 49,
    52, 59, 151–153
Contextualist approach, 48
Coons, Chris, 131
Copenhagen School, 19–21, 23, 27–28,
    31–40, 44, 46, 48–49, 59, 144, 151,
    159, 170

Corry, Olaf, 144, 146, 158
Coulter, Ann, 104
Counterdiscourses, 15
COVID-19 pandemic, 4–5, 30,
    173–177
Crisis decision-making, 18
Critical discourse analysis, 55
Crowley, Candy, 122
Cruz, Ted, 9, 76, 81, 145
Cuomo, Andrew, 9, 25, 82, 120,
    121–124

Dallas Morning News, 122
Dark Continent discourse, 81, 93–94,
    96, 102, 106, 139, 149, 151, 153,
    171
Data gathering, 25–26
Davies, Sara E., 12, 13
de Blasio, Bill, 25, 120
De-exceptionalizing the exception, 51
Derrida, Jacques, 55
Desecuritization, 130–132
de Wilde, Jaap, 19
Dionne, Kim Yi, 94
Discourse analysis, 23–24, 26–27
Discourses. See also individual discourses
    introduction to, 61
    as iterative, 53–54, 55
    multiple, 15–16, 28
    securitizing, 15
    spaces between, 16–17
Discursive approach, 22, 28, 33, 52–58
Discursive sedimentation, 48–49
Dismissal, 112
Dominant signifier, 23–24
Doty, Roxanne Lynn, 37, 45, 54
Drug development, 71
Duncan, Thomas Eric, 9, 16, 113–119,
    120, 121, 124, 133

Economic linkages, 65–66, 67
Elite-centrism, 37, 46, 59
Emergency measures, 19–20, 35–36, 52

Emory University Hospital, 8
Enemark, Christian, 13, 101–102, 169, 177
Eskew, Carter, 126
Exception, the, 21
Exceptionalism. *See also* Schmitt, Carl
   AUT discourse and, 83–84
   as concept, 50–51
   Copenhagen School and, 20–21, 32, 33–34, 37, 46, 48
   defining security and, 144
   expanded concept of, 28
   HWA discourse and, 89–90
   military involvement and, 112–113
   multiple formulations of, 154–155, 157
   Obama and, 107–108
   PGC discourse and, 69–71, 73–74
   potentiality of, 136
   risk and, 146, 155–157
   securitization theory and, 36
Existential threats, 19–20
Expansions, 65
Expertise/expert authority, 17, 29, 72–73, 127, 129, 141–142, 143, 165–168, 174–176
Externalist approach, 44–45

Farenthold, Blake, 79
Farmer, Paul, 89
Fauci, Anthony, 17, 72, 109, 168
"Fear-bola," 2
Fearbola counterdiscourse, 16, 18, 29, 55, 90–96, 118–119, 127–128, 140, 152, 154, 165
Fear of fear, 92, 160
Foreign Policy (magazine), 2–3
Foucault, Michel, 55
Frieden, Thomas, 9, 17, 68, 70, 72, 73, 87, 103–104, 107, 113–114, 116–118, 120, 167, 168
Friend/enemy distinction, 35, 50, 89, 137–139

Garrett, Laurie, 2–3
Gender as performative, 43
Gendered representations, 87
Global circulation, threat of, 68–69
Global health security, 11–15
Global stability, 63, 64–65
Goffman, Erving, 32, 41
Graham, Franklin, 105
Guilfoyle, Kimberly, 123
Gupta, Sanjay, 95, 166

Hagel, Chuck, 131
Hameiri, Shahar, 46
Hansen, Lene, 22, 24, 26, 42–43, 54, 58, 61
Harman, Sophie, 166
Hayes, Chris, 129
Health security as discourse, 168–171
Health-security nexus, 11, 14
Helpless West Africa (HWA) discourse
   audience and, 140
   AUT discourse and, 29, 104–105, 164–165
   containment and, 149
   contestation and, 159
   desecuritization, 16
   Duncan and, 115
   exceptionalism and, 107, 157–158
   Fearbola counterdiscourse and, 91, 95, 154
   Hickox and, 124
   main examination of, 84–90
   midterm elections and, 126
   Obama and, 18, 110
   quarantines and, 122
   racialization and, 171–172
   risk and, 146
   Self/Other relationship and, 137–139
   shifting focus and, 130
   thick meaning of security and, 154
   West African Fragility representation and, 97

Heroic Health Worker, 88, 104, 121,
    123–124, 129, 142, 143
Hickox, Kaci, 2, 9, 93, 122–125, 133,
    142
Higginbottom, Heather, 86
Hindmarch, Suzanne, 46–47
HIV/AIDS, 46–47, 76, 159
Honig, Bonnie, 51
Honigsbaum, Mark, 149
Hot Zone, The (Preston), 79, 95, 152
Human security, 11–12, 13, 84
Huysmans, Jef, 34, 37, 49, 51, 155–156,
    158
Hypothetical Traveler, 106, 121,
    145

Idea theory of securitization, 40
Imagination, 167, 177
Immigration, 37, 45, 152
Indispensable Nation, 73, 78, 84, 88, 92,
    111, 137, 151
Influenza, 76–77
Intensity, 51
Intertextuality, 58, 62, 79, 94–95
Isakson, John, 67

Jasanoff, Sheila, 168, 176
Johnson, Jeh, 115–116
Jones, Lee, 46

Kaplan, Robert, 177
Kelly, John F., 80
Kerry, John, 73, 85
Key events, concept of, 58, 100
Kidjo, Angelique, 128, 143
Kim, Jim Yong, 89
Klain, Ron, 9, 71–72, 118
Kristeva, Julia, 58

Larson, Heidi J., 168
Leander, Anna, 167
Léonard, Sarah, 20, 23, 32, 40
Liberalism of fear, 160

Liu, Joanne, 8, 88, 107–108, 130
Lobo-Guerrero, Luis, 144

Maddow, Rachel, 94
McDonald, Matt, 39
McInnes, Colin, 159
Médecins Sans Frontières, 8, 9, 85, 88,
    107, 110, 121, 130
Media
    AUT discourse and, 74, 79
    Fearbola counterdiscourse and, 93,
        127
    HWA discourse and, 85
    PGC discourse and, 65, 67, 72–73
    role of, 37
Meet the Press, 108, 109
Merlin, Toby, 79
Midterm elections, 10, 125–128, 132,
    133, 140
Military involvement, 8, 70, 88, 109,
    111, 112–113, 131, 152
Model 2, 24, 26
Multiplicity, 23, 32, 45, 55
Mutation, threat of, 68–69, 77, 109–
    110, 111–112

National Institutes of Health, 130
National security, 11, 12–14
Neal, Andrew W., 21
Neglect, 149–150
Neo-Marxism, 32
New York Times, 109
Nodal point, 23
Nossiter, Adam, 85, 88
Nunes, João, 149

Obama, Barack
    audience and, 44
    AUT discourse and, 111–112
    authority and, 143
    criticism of, 115, 118, 126
    exceptionalism and, 107
    on fear, 92

Fearbola counterdiscourse and, 95
Friedan and, 117–118
funding requests from, 10, 126–127, 130–131
HWA discourse and, 85, 110
military involvement and, 88
PGC discourse and, 63, 64–65, 68, 69–70, 71–74, 109, 110, 112
political motivation of, 2
quarantines and, 3
on response as "self-interest," 18
risk and, 145
securitizing moves of, 108–113, 116
shifting focus and, 130
speeches of, 1, 8, 132, 154, 163
"success" and, 131–132
timing of response and, 147
travel bans and, 9, 168
O'Connell, Stephen, 86
Ontological gerrymandering, 42, 45
Operation United Assistance, 8, 109
O'Reilly, Bill, 114
Osterholm, Michael, 68, 109, 111, 175
Othering, 87, 89, 90, 94, 102, 124, 128, 135–136, 138, 164. *See also* Self/ Other relationship
Ouamouno, Emile, 6
Outbreak, 79, 152
Outbreak, representations of, 101–102
Outbreak narrative, 17, 78–79, 152, 174

Paris School, 21, 22, 32, 37–38, 46, 51
Paul, Rand, 80
Performativity, 43
Pham, Nina, 9, 116–117, 129, 133
Pharmaceuticals
  Magic Bullet of, 71, 83, 84, 88–89, 169
  safety testing in, 112
Play of practice, 58
Political construction of disease, 14
Poststructuralism, 22, 32, 33, 42–43, 45, 54–56, 59

"Post-truth" politics, 18
Potential Global Catastrophe (PGC) discourse
  airport screenings and, 82
  audience and, 140
  AUT discourse and, 29, 79, 116, 129–130, 164
  authority and, 141
  containment and, 149
  contestation and, 159
  desecuritization, 16
  Duncan and, 113, 115
  exceptionalism and, 155, 157–158
  expertise and, 129
  Fearbola counterdiscourse and, 91, 95
  HWA discourse and, 88, 90
  main examination of, 63–74
  midterm elections and, 125, 128
  Obama and, 18, 109, 110, 112, 131
  outbreak narrative and, 78, 152
  quarantines and, 122
  risk and, 144–145, 145–146
  Self/Other relationship and, 137–139
  West African Fragility representation and, 97
Potentiality versus immediacy, 63
Predication, 57–58
Preston, Richard, 79, 152
Presupposition, 57, 67
Process, securitization as, 158–160
Public Health Emergency of International Concern, 8

Quammen, David, 102
Quarantines, 9–10, 17, 81–83, 89, 121–124, 143
Questions for analysis, 54

Racialization, 171–172
Reagan, Ronald, 176
Realism, 32
Referent objects, 19–20, 35–36, 63, 64, 75–77, 85, 86–88

Relevant audience, 19–20
Rice, Susan, 73
Risk/risk studies, 37–38, 51, 103, 135–
     136, 144–146, 155–158
Roe, Paul, 41
Rushton, Simon, 159
Ruzicka, Jan, 20, 23, 32, 40

Salia, Martin, 128, 129
Salter, Mark, 41
Samaritan's Purse, 8, 85, 105
SARS, 76
Schmitt, Carl, 21, 28, 34–35, 37, 46,
     50–51, 59, 138, 155. *See also*
     Exceptionalism
"Scientization of politics," 176
Securitization as process, 52
Securitization theory, 13–14, 19–23,
     27, 31, 33–40, 35, 57, 58–59, 136,
     170
Securitizing actors, 19–20, 35–36, 41,
     43, 47–48, 92–93
Securitizing moves, 35, 41–42, 53,
     108–113
Securitizing speech acts, 19–20, 108
Security, meaning and logic of, 1–2, 48–
     52, 101
Sedimentation argument, 34–35
Self, construction of, 75
Self/Other relationship, 100–101, 124,
     132, 135, 137–139, 151, 164. *See
     also* Othering
Shaheen, Jeanne, 125
Shklar, Judith, 91, 92, 160
Siegel, Marc, 72, 166
Signifiers, 23–24
Simmet, Hilton R., 168, 176
Slaven, Mike, 37
Smith, Christopher, 106, 138
Snyderman, Nancy, 166
Social constructivism, 32
Social media, 24–25
Sociological school/model, 20, 21, 32

Song, Weiqing, 55
Sovereign, power of, 37
Spanish flu, 78
Speculation, 114
Speech acts
     audience and, 41, 47–48
     as embedded within social context,
         44
     securitization theory and, 34, 35, 36,
         38, 39
Spencer, Craig, 3, 9, 25, 119–122, 124,
     129
State breakdown, threat of, 66–68
Stritzel, Holger, 39, 41, 44, 47, 54–55,
     141
Subject-positioning, 57–58, 67, 72, 75,
     94, 123–124, 129
Survival, security's meaning and, 34
Systems of signification, 23–24

Temporality, 63
Texas Health Presbyterian Hospital, 9
Thickness, security's, 153–154
Thick signifiers, 49
Threat perception, shifting, 129
Threats, 63, 64, 66–67, 109, 111–112
Trade restrictions, lack of, 70
Transgression, 51–52
Travel bans, 9, 10, 17, 70, 81–83, 95,
     168
Treatment disparity, 105
Treatment units, 10
Trump, Donald, 104, 173, 174, 176

Uncertainty, 79–80, 135, 167, 174–
     175
United Nations (UN), 108, 109, 154,
     169
USAID, 1, 6, 8, 10, 25, 107, 147
US Department of Defense, 1, 6, 8, 25,
     108, 147
US Department of Homeland Security,
     airport screenings and, 9

US House Subcommittee on Africa, Global Health, Global Human Rights, and International Organizations, 103–104, 111, 117
US Senate Committee on Appropriations, 86

Valued referent objects, 35–36
van Munster, Rens, 51, 144, 167
van Rythoven, Eric, 45
Varga, Daniel, 117
Vaughn, Jocelyn, 41
Vernacular security, 151
Vinson, Amber Joy, 9, 116–117, 129, 133
Vulnerability, 52
Vuori, Juha A., 41

Wæver, Ole, 19, 32–33, 35, 40, 49, 52, 55, 59, 144–145, 146, 155, 167
Wald, Priscilla, 78, 151–152
Washington Post, 123–124
Weir, Lorna, 13
Wenham, Clare, 14, 166, 169
West African Fragility representation, 67–68, 74, 78, 80–81, 84, 86, 90, 97, 102, 128, 137–138
WHO, 8, 105, 110, 112, 168
Wilhemsen, Julie, 42–43, 55
Williams, Bisa, 66
Williams, Michael C., 22, 34, 37, 42, 91, 160
Women, invisibility of, 166
World Bank, 89
Writebol, Nancy, 8, 73, 102–108, 111, 121, 133, 142, 148

Zakaria, Fareed, 95